Praise for "The Cancer Challenge: Sharing the Experience"

"A fascinating look into the beginnings of the self-help movement for breast cancer. The fascinating story of how women coped with this disease seen through the experience and eyes of one woman's journey from patient to educator during her successful struggle against breast cancer and the ignorance surrounding a diagnosis of cancer in the 1970's."

Richard Shapiro, MD FACS
Associate Professor of Surgery
NYU Clinical Cancer Institute
NYU School of Medicine

"Lee Miller speaks from the voice of authenticity and experience in turning what is typically a negative personal health issue into help and hope for so many others through SHARE.
She is a leader in the self-help movement helping people to see the value and benefit of the collective wisdom of experiential expertise. Anyone facing a chronic disease who desires to get back control can benefit from Lee's wisdom in "The Cancer Challenge: Sharing the Experience.""

Amye L. Leong MBA
President & CEO, Healthy Motivation
International Spokesperson, United Nations Bone and Joint Decade 2000-2010 Former Chair, U.S. Surgeon General's National Council on Self-Help & Public Health

"SHARE has helped countless women take back control of their lives after receiving the diagnosis of cancer. Lee's accounts form a compelling and worthy testimony to both the heart of these individual women and the power of the groups they form."

David L. Stevens, MD
Assistant Professor of Medicine
New York University School of Medicine
Director, Department of Medicine
Gouverneur Healthcare Services

# The Cancer Challenge: Sharing the Experience

# The Cancer Challenge: Sharing the Experience

*Lee Miller*

iUniverse, Inc.
New York  Lincoln  Shanghai

## The Cancer Challenge: Sharing the Experience

iUniverse books may be ordered through booksellers or by contacting:

iUniverse
2021 Pine Lake Road, Suite 100
Lincoln, NE 68512
www.iuniverse.com
1-800-Authors (1-800-288-4677)

ISBN: 978-0-595-42981-3 (pbk)
ISBN: 978-0-595-87322-7 (ebk)

Printed in the United States of America

# Dedication

How does one begin to acknowledge all of the people who have been part of SHARE? We would have to go back to 1976 and mention all of the pioneers who sculpted the form this support group would take. Breaking new ground, giving up time and energy to help it expand and ultimately reach thousands of people. Giving real meaning to the term "peer support." We cannot measure inspiration and courage; we can be guided by them and use them to forge ahead.

There have been many who have not lived to witness SHARE approach its thirtieth year of existence. But their spirit and commitment remain deep in the recesses of our history, and have altered us and helped to create our present identity.

There are numerous volunteers upon whose shoulders we have helped to build our structure: the facilitators, the hotline volunteers, the telephone calls and mailings that had to be done in order to exist. There are those who attended conferences and brought back their learnings to us and helped educate us about cancer. They were always there and they will always be here. We now have a paid staff of twelve. Each supervises a program with her own expertise; their contributions cannot be measured. They are the core and crux of all the programs of which we are so proud.

The word "sisterhood" has often been used casually. But at SHARE, it is a reality. Those who visit our office feel the special quality and so this book is dedicated to all of the women in SHARE who teach us that coping is courage and that looking into the abyss enhances the blue of the sky.

# Contents

# Special Thanks

I would be remiss if I did not give special thanks to my dear children, their spouses and my grandchildren for the love and support they have always provided for me. This has given me the strength to combat some of life's challenges and the incentive to write this book. Once again, the value of connection has been demonstrated to me and provides the core component in helping me to face life's struggles whether it be career choices or cancer.

I also wish to include my dear friends (you know who you are) who are truly family.

And a big hug to Mitchell for helping me with my computer challenges.

# Preface

Early in the winter of 1968, S.J., a twenty year old New York University student, came to the Breast Disease Clinic at the PMI-Strang Clinic because of a pea sized nodule in the upper outer quadrant of her left breast. Both her physical examination and mammogram didn't reveal any suspicious characteristics. In addition, she had no other history of "risk factors" and finally, because her age put her in the lowest possible "probability category" for development of Breast Cancer, no biopsy was recommended. Nevertheless, pursuant to the Breast Disease Clinic protocol for the follow-up of any newly discovered, first, discrete breast lesion, she was scheduled for quarterly re-evaluations over the next twelve months.

On the third post discovery re-examination, the only change was minimal skin dimpling over the nodule. Though the repeat mammogram was again reported as "negative", a biopsy was performed and the nodule was found to be malignant. S. J. was discharged from the hospital. In addition to awaiting a comprehensive analysis of the biopsy specimen, she was scheduled for a complete physical assessment and metastatic work-up.

For the next three months S. J. seemed to have vanished. She failed to keep her appointments, didn't contact the Clinic and didn't respond to phone messages. When she finally returned, she was in tears and obviously depressed. She said she felt isolated and alone. She related that when she tried to discuss her "problem" with her female peers, the first and only question that they asked was "are you pregnant?" It was as if this were the only significant tragedy that could occur in a young woman's life! She also felt that she couldn't discuss this with any male friends or male family members. Her depression led her to break off a relationship with her boyfriend; led her to feel that she would be physically unattractive and could never have children, or a career It led her to isolation from school, family and friends.

My medical practice at the time, was exclusively in the area of breast diseases and over the next six to seven years I treated approximately twenty-five women under the age of thirty-five years. Each of them exhibited the same emotional and psychological reaction that I observed in S.J., but in varying degrees of intensity. All women, regardless of age, who are diagnosed with breast cancer will experience some degree of depression, anger because of physical changes, fear for the future and isolation. Nevertheless, it became clear to me that young women, those under the age of 35 years, are faced with some unique circumstances that most women above that age are less likely to encounter.

Most individuals, men and women in the age group under thirty-five years are more likely to be in the "creation" phase of their lives. They are in school preparing for the future; starting families or watching their young children grow; beginning and developing jobs and careers. It is well known that this age group is probably least likely to be thinking about saving money, particularly for retirement. Few in this age group have suffered life threatening illness or injuries. Also, they are the least likely to have suffered the loss of friends, siblings, parents, or even grandparents as a result of injuries or disease. If an individual in this age group contracts a life threatening illness, they would have difficulty finding peer group support, experience or understanding.

With these realizations in mind, I looked around and found that there were no organizations set up to address the concerns of these women in an ongoing way. The American Cancer Society had a program, in Manhattan at least, called "Reach for Recovery". At a physician's request only, a woman who had a mastectomy visits the patient in the hospital, usually a few days after the surgery. The primary purpose of the visit is to attempt to reassure the patient that she can look good and continue to lead a normal life. In the '60's and '70's this program didn't offer any follow-up visits for the patient, nor were any other services provided. It was essentially limited to "Look at me! If I can make it, so can you. Further, if the visit weren't specifically requested by the patient's physician, then there could be no knowledge about, or access to the patient …

I thought that more was needed! I spoke with several women on the Board of Trustees for PMI-Strang Clinic about this concern and my desire to attempt starting a "discussion" group for these women. The medical director, Dr. Daniel Miller, and the Board gave their approval and support for the project. Buffy Cobb, a prominent member of both the community and the Strang Board, arranged for me to be interviewed by her good friend, Miss Arlene Francis, on her "talk-radio" program. Miss Francis was the Bill Moyers of radio in her day and explored topical issues and events through probing questions of her guests. Her program was aired five days a week at mid morning on station WOR and the broadcast reached Greater Metropolitan New York, Connecticut and Long Island.

In late July of 1976, I was interviewed by Miss Francis on her show. We discussed some of the current issues about Breast Cancer diagnosis and treatment, but we spent most of the interview on the emotional burden of this disease. My recollection of this interview is that we discussed this for all women and not just for young women. At the end of the interview I announced that in two weeks there would be a meeting at Strang Clinic and that all women who had Breast Cancer, or who had had a mastectomy, would be welcomed. We gave the date, day and time. They were told that no advance registration or reservation would be needed and that there would be no charge. The topic would be their experience surrounding the diagnosis, treatment and post-treatment of their breast cancer.

When the day arrived and the hour approached for the meeting, I had no idea if anyone would show up, or if there would be a crowd. The Clinic had received a few calls about the meeting, but no records were kept and there was no indication if the callers intended to come … At 6:00 PM, the hour of the meeting a dozen women had shown up and SHARE was born.

The next four years were fascinating. Meetings were held at least every month, and sometimes bi-monthly. Though I have no attendance records at this time, there frequently were many more than a dozen women attending the meetings and other events. Over this period many issues were explored and included the effects of the disease on children, spouses, significant others and sexuality; clothing, prosthesis and reconstructive surgery; pregnancy, radiation therapy, chemotherapy and alternative medicine; job and insurance discrimination; and last, but not least, their treating physicians and their medical care. Most gratifying, was the fact that the women gradually evolved into a true "peer support" group.

My role in this group rapidly became that of an advisor and the "medical face" both of the group and for the group. I was fully accepted in all of the discussions, regardless of the topic. I was the proverbial "fly on the wall"

In retrospect, note that SHARE was founded at a time early in the "self-help" and "peer support" movement in this country. This is particularly true as it applies to groups organizing around specific diseases. SHARE also continues to be unique in the fact that it took up the cause of ovarian cancer, a related disease, and has added relevant programs to the same principles and programs models. SHARE continues to be primarily an organization with minimum paid professional staff and with most programs facilitated by volunteers. It is unique in that it is a disease oriented voluntary organization that is also multilingual, has been invited to foreign countries to demonstrate the "peer support" model and has been participating in the training of medical residents at a major hospital and medical school in Manhattan on how to communicate with cancer patients and their families.

I'm proud to say that I founded SHARE, but I'm more proud of the many women whose labor, vision, commitment and guidance developed the organization from its "bare bones" beginning to the level of professionalism that marks its services today

Dr. Eugene Thiessen

# Introduction

Once you have been diagnosed with cancer, you enter another world. You have ceased having the illusion of control over your own body. Some unknown intruder has invaded you, and you are at its mercy. Even when you seem to be doing well (all the tests are good) there is the hovering shadow of death over you, and any new blip such as a headache or swollen finger may portend for you the return of this intruder. You never feel quite safe and the periods between medical visits give you some surcease but the fear can be awakened at any moment. Often, when you wake up in the morning, your first thought is about the fact that you have cancer now and you have been unalterably changed in a way that precludes the old YOU from ever returning.

You begin to look at the world in a different way, and evaluate how you spend your time in this very finite life; how are you being treated by others? You begin to understand the difference between sympathy and empathy. The former makes you feel diminished and the latter understood.

Perhaps you make new plans, doing things you never would have done before. Now is the chance, you feel, perhaps the only chance you will ever have. Some changes are very positive; the step you delayed before has become more urgent now, and you want to fill your life with meaning

You become more sensitive to the treatment you receive from others; it is easy to feel rejected when you did not receive the telephone calls or offers of support you expected and needed. You are not ready to forgive or understand that fear or one's inability to cope are often the reasons others have deserted you in this time of need. You feel abandoned!

You also begin to love with consciousness You realize the importance of your relationships, and you appreciate the support being given. Your time is a valuable commodity and you do not wish to squander it with people with whom you no longer wish to spend time You understand that time is NOT infinite. You have been robbed of your innocence; you finally understand that facing the possibility of death means losing your feeling of invulnerablity. But, facing reality can enhance the good times, change your perspective and establish your priorities. You become able to ask the question "If not now, when?" The social hypocrisy that most of us indulge in from time to time seems superfluous. Living with uncertainty is difficult, but it is possible. Having cancer has taught us what was always true, that life is uncertain.

Hopefully, the following pages will give credence to these ideas and illustrate how we handle the challenge of cancer.

# My Story

In 1975, <u>MZ</u> magazine printed an article about breast cancer It talked about breast self-examination. It mentioned that if you raised your arm and you felt a lump and the area around it dimpled or wrinkled, it probably was malignant. I had given my husband the article to read that night.

Later, that night, I did a self-exam and felt a slight protuberance, and when I raised my arm, the area around it did dimple.

I ran into the living room where my husband was sitting and had him feel the area on my breast where I had felt the protrusion. It was very small, and he said he could not feel anything. Then, I raised my arm and the area dimpled and his face grew very pale and I knew at that moment that I HAD BREAST CANCER1

Nine days later, I was admitted to the hospital for a biopsy or a mastectomy, depending upon what they found. That morning, I was wheeled into the waiting area on a gurney awaiting my turn to have the surgery. I was slightly fuzzy due to some pre-operative sedative they had given me, but the enormity of the situation took hold of me. As I lay there waiting, I stroked my left breast and said "goodbye" to it The significance of the situation struck me and I wondered how I could live without my breast.

As I lay on the operating table, the surgeon came in wearing a green surgical outfit Because of my medicated state, I thought he was a knight riding in to rescue me, and I yelled out "It's the left!" The next thing I remember was that I was lying in bed with my chest wrapped in a bandage, and I was told I had undergone a radical mastectomy. I thought the word "radical" referred to a political party. The good news was that there was no nodal involvement. I had no idea what the implications were of all of this, but I felt that death was probably imminent This was 1975 and at that time cancer was often thought to be a prelude to death.

I began to think of how I would change my life if I had only six months to live, and I decided to keep it the way it was; I loved my family, friends and my job and I did not wish to travel around the world or take myself away from my life. I did not know then that a new journey would begin with my participation in SHARE, and that my life would be changed forever!

# 1

# The Beginning (We are more alike than different)

SHARE was born on August 1976, one week after a hurricane delayed our first meeting. Perhaps this was a portent of things to come—a violent wrenching of wind and rain stirring up and pouring out of emotions and unpredictable outcomes. At that time there was little recognition of the need for psycho-social and emotional support for us, the breast cancer survivors.

The meeting was called by Dr. Eugene Thiessen, a concerned breast specialist who noted that there was an increase in the number of women in their twenties being diagnosed with breast cancer. He felt that they needed peers to talk to, since the majority of women diagnosed with breast cancer were in their forties and fifties. The meeting was advertised over the radio in an interview with Arlene Frances and Dr. Thiessen. When I heard the announcement, I was thrilled that I would meet with others who had been through the same experience as I. Although I was in my forties at that time, there was no barrier to my attending.

I myself had a radical mastectomy on Jan. 28, 1975 at 2:35 PM. I remember clearly being frightened and trembling, because at that time, a diagnosis of breast cancer was viewed as certain death. Also, the treatment of lumpectomies, followed by radiation, was not being practiced then, so the loss of a breast and the possibility of death presented a double tribulation. I will not use the word "challenge", since ignorance of the disease and the notion that nothing much could be done to save one, overcame a more positive outlook.

My size 36B had always been a matter of some pride to me and the feeling that part of my body had been amputated made me feel damaged.

When you lose a part of your anatomy, there is a feeling of loss and incompleteness and sometimes disgust and rejection of your body. One of the women I met in the hospital was so repelled by her own body-image that she refused to touch the area, even when she showered she would not wash the area. Finally, it became so dirty that the doctor insisted that she clean it.

At that time, a woman would remain in the hospital for several days after a mastectomy. During those days, I learned that I had no nodal involvement and that no further treatment was necessary. I did not understand enough about the disease to realize that I had received good news. Of course, this did not keep me from my belief that the disease would kill me. For many months I woke up in the middle of the night; even my husband's arms wrapped protectively around me did not minimize my fears.

One late afternoon at the hospital, a meeting was called for the breast cancer patients and their partners. Also attending was a couple where the woman had previously had a mastectomy. They were invited to speak about their relationship. He had met her after her mastectomy; they met, fell in love and married. She was wearing a turtle-neck sweater and her bosom looked perfectly normal (this was in the days before reconstruction).Her husband told us that the absence of a breast only made her dearer to him. These were such encouraging words, because at that time having only one breast felt like a terrible deformity and represented a loss of femininity to many of us. That meeting probably gave me my first glimpse of how helpful and comfortable it could be to speak to other women with breast cancer.

One year later, Dr. Eugene Thiessen turned that dream into a reality! Twelve women were present at that first meeting and we sat in a circle in a room at Strang Clinic where Dr.Thiessen worked. His wife, Ina was there graciously serving coffee to all of us and it was not until the next meeting that we decided that only those with breast cancer could attend. We had a tremendous sense of privacy and exclusionary feelings towards those who were "civilians" in our army of "breast cancer survivors." The disease made us feel diminished both physically and mentally.

And so, the meeting began … Twelve women and Dr. Thiessen sat in a circle and as we looked at each other, tears of relief filled our eyes. We knew that each of us understood viscerally what effect the disease had on us. What we were beginning to learn was that although we were strangers, we all had much in common—a crushing life-altering realization that death might claim us in the not-to-distant future. Perhaps, for the first time in our lives, we had to come to grips with our own mortality: death left the realm of the theoretical.

The idea that the commonality of experience could help us to explore, examine and face the challenge of living with cancer was born that evening. It became the root and core of SHARE. We slowly evolved out of the needs of our membership and developed into a grass-roots organization. It was a slow and arduous process, but exciting too because it was a way to seize control over our lives; something the disease had made us feel was impossible.

Dr. Thiessen facilitated the first group and it was suggested that someone with mental health experience might co-facilitate, since there would be many emotional issues which would emerge. I slowly raised my hand and volunteered, since I had the requisite experience and had been diagnosed in 1975, about a year before most of the others in the group.

Everyone was delighted to be relieved of this responsibility, and they applauded when 1 accepted. I felt I had been awarded a gold cup. For the first time in a year, I realized that something positive could be pulled out of this horrendous situation.

We talked of our fears, our shame (yes, shame) because we suddenly felt like outsiders in a world of non-cancer people. Some of us felt we were going crazy, but we soon learned that we were not alone, and our feelings were not unique. Although we were all different people with different personalities, there was a universality in our feelings, although we handled them differently.

We also initiated an exercise in order to help overcome our repugnant feelings about the empty site which a breast had once occupied. It involved looking in a mirror, stroking the empty place and concentrating on the fact that this was our new body, and it belonged to us and therefore, was special.

I tried this daily for many weeks, and finally became more accustomed to my altered self. It did not preclude embarrassment, however, when I was without the prosthesis and someone saw me.

At that first meeting we sat in a circle looking into each other's eyes, and began to speak about our fear of dying. In 1976, a diagnosis of breast cancer was equivalent to a death sentence. We had feelings of inadequacy and loss of femininity, due to the amputation of a breast. Mastectomies were the prevailing treatment at that time.

We asked, "what did they do with the breast we lost in the operating room? Did they discard it after studying it? Was it in the garbage bin?" Would we ever date again? How would we tell the new person in our lives that we had only one breast or sometimes none?

Tears of relief flooded our eyes as others nodded in understanding and we realized we were not alone. We felt we were now different from the rest of the population. Would we ever feel "normal" again? How could we keep our families from worrying about us, and thus maximizing our own fears? We were living with a sense of doom: waiting for a shoe to fall.

It felt so good to be able to verbalize these feelings; we felt only those who had been through this experience could truly understand.

In 1976, the only organization dealing with breast cancer was the American Cancer Society. They did not have group support then, but had "Reach to Recovery" volunteers visit us in the hospital and give us a small stocking stuffed with a piece of soft material which acted as a prosthesis, since the area after the surgery was too tender to accommodate anything firmer.

It takes a long time to really form a sisterhood: a core of women who trust each other, discuss their innermost thoughts and feelings and really LISTEN to each other and nod their heads in affirmation. But, in a relatively short time, perhaps because of the severity of the disease and the fear of death hovering overhead, we managed to coalesce and build friendships. When one of the women refused to have any surgery or chemotherapy despite a very negative prognosis regarding her recovery, the group jumped on her in anger, because they were worried about her.

As a facilitator, it was my responsibility to intervene and explain that she had done her exploration and had made her own decision. The only thing the woman wanted to do was to control her own nutrition. She was unable to purchase a pressure cooker which she felt was necessary, because of financial constraints. The woman in the group who had been angriest at her during the meeting because she felt that rejecting chemotherapy in some way negated her own choice of treatment, brought in a pressure cooker for her at the next meeting. So, although we did not always agree, provided there was enough information for someone to make a choice, we respected the autonomy of each individual. We also knew that an uninformed decision is not a valid decision.

We named our organization "S.H.A.R.E.". It stood for "self-help action and rap experience." At that time, the word "rap" was used to mean "talking, chatting, and it often described the kind of conversation that went on in support groups.

## The "C" Word

It was not too long ago when euphemisms were used to say that someone had died of cancer It was often called "a long-standing disease." Obituary notices rarely mentioned the WORD. So, naturally, it is not surprising that a great deal of shame was attached to having the disease. What a relief to sit with a group of women and use all of the real terms such as "mastectomy," "chemo-therapy," "radiation," and "metastases"

Each of us began to tell our story. The details of finding the lump, seeing the doctor, the fear, the terror of hearing the word "cancer", the denial, the anger the disbelief some or all of these feelings were expressed by all.

Almost all of the women had undergone mastectomies; they were still the rule of the day, despite the fact that lumpectomies with radiation were now gaining popularity. There was so much shame … feeling like a "freak" with one breast. Going into a locker room was a problem; concealing yourself while you undressed. We also began to use the words "breast cancer" when asked about our illness. We began to feel that we must educate the public, that our attitude and honesty would help reduce our shame and teach others that cancer could become part of the language without drawing looks of horror and pity. Sometimes we laughed as when one of the women told how she had been swimming in the Carribean with a new man she had met. Her prosthesis slipped down into the lower part of her bathing suit, and she was trying to pull it back up without being seen by her companion. She tugged and tugged and finally managed to do it. Later, when talking to a friend who had been observing them from the beach, she confessed her embarrassment and her friend said "Don't worry, while you were doing that he was trying to get his testicles back into his suit"

Another woman who had belonged to a nudist colony, told how after her mastectomy, she wore a towel draped around her torso because she felt ashamed of having only one breast When the other people saw her covered up, they formed a circle around her, hugged her and told her to remove the towel; they loved her just the way she was. She reluctantly took off the towel with tears in her eyes and began the difficult lesson of learning that she was still the same person regardless of the number of breasts she had.

Years later, a very courageous woman posed for the N.Y Times Magazine section with her chest bare and a flower tattoo over her chest where a breast had once resided. We were thrilled and encouraged by this act.

As we began to know each other better, our guard lessened and we began to explore in more depth our innermost feelings. One of the women discussed a date with a new boyfriend. When the evening ended and they were planning a sexual interlude, she felt it was time she told him about her mastectomy. So, first she took a shower, wrapped herself in a bathrobe, came out, took a deep breath and said "I have something to tell you." He said, "I am a doctor and you gave me many clues. It makes no difference to me." We all heaved a sigh of relief and decided that acceptance of that fact differentiated the men from the boys. Of course, it wasn't as easy as that and we had some conversations and role-playing on when to tell and how to tell.

The seventies was a time of change. Mastectomies were becoming much less common; reconstruction was in vogue. Attitudes of patients were changing. The Women's Movement gave rise to an assertion that patients needed to have a say in their treatment. The Doctor was being removed from his/her pedestal, and the fear of asking questions or obtaining a second opinion was diminishing.

In March of 1977, a woman named Jackie Bleiberg applied for a job at Saks Fifth Avenue department store. She had been offered the job, but the offer was withdrawn after she told the store's nurse that she had undergone a mastectomy in November. The National Organization for Women organized a protest and picket line in front of Saks. Many SHARE women participated and cut up their Saks charge cards. The picketers marched in a circle in front of the store during the lunch hour, chanting "Don't shop at Saks. This store discriminates against women." Photographers were present. The New York Times printed the article and the protest was shown on TV that evening. Shortly, thereafter, the store's chairman and chief executive officer apologized and offered Ms. Bleiberg a job, which she refused. She said later, "I opened up a Pandora's box for other women and I am glad I did it How many other cases are there like mine that you don't hear about because the other women are too embarrassed to come forward?"

In that same year, 1977, SHARE incorporated as a not-for-profit organization staffed exclusively by volunteers.

## Protesters Assail Refusal of Saks to Hire Woman after Mastectomy

New York Times 3/25/77

Twenty women cut their Saks Fifth Avenue charge cards` into pieces in front of the Fifth Avenue store yesterday to protest the stores recent refusal to hire a woman who had had a cancerous breast removed. The demonstrators also urged shoppers to boycott the store.

Although the store has since notified the woman, Jacqueline Bleiberg of Bayside, Queens, that she can have the $140 a week job, selling handbags, "any time she wants it," she took part in the demonstration yesterday.

Later yesterday, Allan R. Johnson, the store's chairman and chief executive officer apologized to Mrs. Bleiberg "for the way this whole thing was-handled."

"It was a mistake," he said in a meeting with a group of the de nonstraxors in his office. "Our interviewer did not follow the procedure of asking the woman to get an opinion from her doctor on whether she can do the job.

Mr. Johnson repeated the store's offer that Mrs. Bleiberg could come to work at Safs whenever she wanted to, but she told him she still felt "too devastated" to consider the offer.

"My doctor had told me I was absolute ly free of cancer, and he gave me no restrictions," she told Mr. Johnson. "So you can imagine how I felt when. I walked out of your personnel office last week."

Mrs. Bleiberg said later that she was considering taking legal action a gainst the store.

"I opened up a Pandora's box for other women, and I'm glad I did it," she said angrily. "How many other cases are there like mine that you don't hear about, be cause the women are too embarrassed to come forward?"

The protesters, many of them wearing expensive fur coat, marched in a circle in front of the store during the lunch hour, chanting: "Don't shop it Saks, don't shop at Saks, this store discriminates against women."

They included members of the National Organization for Women, as well as former mastectomy patients who belong to a Manhattan troup called the Post Mastectomy Discussion Group, organized by Dr. Eugene Thiessen, a breast cancer specialist.

Mrs. Bleiberg, who was recently dlvorcedk said that she had been offered the job last Tuesday, but that the offer was withdrawn after she told the store's nurse that she bad had a mastectomy in November.

Mrs. Beeiberg said that when she demanded to know why she could not have the job, she was told by a personnel interviewer: "I'm sorry, but we have to go by our rules."

In some respects, we saw ourselves as educators; being more public about our condition and helping to dispel the idea of "cancer victim", instead, presenting the idea of a full human being who happens to have cancer. But of course we had to convince ourselves of that first. We were able to do that through the solidarity and coping mechanisms established in the group. Our meeting place was a sanctuary; a place where we felt at home and understood. We learned the value of each day, and many of us made plans for our lives which we would not have made before the disease. One woman got a divorce, another moved to Arizona. These were desires we had previously toyed with but had never put into effect until we understood that life is finite and we owed it to ourselves to lead the most fulfilling lives we could. We learned the difference between selfishness and enlightened self-interest. We did not know how much time we had, but we wanted it to be quality time.

## Quality and Quanity

In the final analysis, which is more important to us, quality of life or longevity? Some would say the answer seems evident; of course we want to be able to live as fully as possible, but what about those for whom the extra time, albeit pain-ridden and uncomfortable, means seeing a new grandchild or mending fences with a family member or friend? How much more treatment must we endure? Is it really worth it? Only the person involved can truly decide; our value systems are individual and what we deem most important is based on our life experience. Others cannot make the decision for us as long as we have mental capacity; the decision is our own. We who stand by and watch need to support fully the wishes of the patient But with this addendum, that the person making the decision is aware of all the options and consequences.

This is a most difficult time for all, but respecting the integrity of the individual making the choice is paramount, and inherent in that decision is a lesson for many of life's quandaries.

We begin to look at the world in a different way, and to evaluate how we spent our time in this very finite life. How were we being treated by others? We began to understand the difference between sympathy and empathy. The former makes you feel diminished and the latter understood Perhaps we made new plans doing things we would never have done before. Now was the chance and perhaps the only chance we would ever have. Some of the changes were very positive; the step we delayed before became more urgent now and we wanted to fill our lives with meaning. We became more sensitive to the treatment we received from others; it was easy to feel rejected when we did not receive the telephone calls or offers of support we expected and needed. We were not ready to forgive or understand that fear or inability to cope were the reasons others had deserted us in this time of need. We felt abandoned!

We also began to love with consciousness, with awareness of the importance of relationships and appreciation for the support being given. Our time was a valuable commodity and we did not wish to squander it with people with whom we no longer wished to spend time. We understood that time is **NOT** infinite. We had been robbed of our innocence. We finally understood that facing the possibility of death means losing our feeling of invulnerablity. But facing reality can enhance the good times, change one's perspective and establish priorities. We became able to ask the question, "If not now, when? "The social hypocrisy most of us indulge in from time to time seemed superfluous. Living with uncertainty is difficult but it is possible. Having cancer taught us what was always true; that life is uncertain.

As the year passed, we formed another group co-led by two facilitators. Training took place by listening to the tape of the meeting and discussing this with the facilitators. The participants in the group had consented to this procedure. Word of mouth attracted many more to our meetings, and by 1977, we became a not-for-profit organization staffed exclusively by volunteers. We began to meet in other places wherever we could secure free space. We distributed notices of our meetings with our physicians, and in hospitals and in public places where we thought we might reach interested people.

We also put in place a more sophisticated training program for our facilitators and hotline volunteers. Other organizations were calling us for advice on how to proceed with their breast cancer organizations. We were happy to share what we had learned and are pleased today that many of these groups incorporated our suggestions and are now very successful.

Our distinctive feature *is* peer support, which means that our facilitators and hotline volunteers are cancer survivors themselves, thus adding the dimension of their own experience as well as their expertise. We are fond of saying "experience is our expertise."

Our support groups kept growing and there were requests for many different types of groups, such as one for those undergoing chemo-therapy, one for the newly diagnosed, for single women, and for caregiving and family groups and wellness programs.

All of our records were kept under the bed of our Secretary.

*originally published as a My Turn column in the November 29, 1976 issue of Newsweek. 9A*

MY Turn

## Cancer is Not a Four-Letter Word

## By Nina Diamond

-

When the doctor said those awful words, "The biopsied node is malignant, you have cancer," the world didn't come to an end or even stop for a brief moment Everything went on as usual, but somehow nothing would ever be as before for me. Some of the changes would be for the better, as my feeling for life intensified.

I discovered that cancer is not a four-letter word, though just saying it befouls the air because of our fear of the disease. Cancer strikes one out of every four people, which means one around every bridge table, in a golf foursome or in a set of tennis doubles. The reality of cancer is something I've had to learn to live with anew each' day.

For me it all began when I turned over in bed one night, and felt a searing pain under my arm. Further investigation during my shower the following morning disclosed a lump nestled comfortably in a bed of tissue between the upper breast and armpit. My immediate reaction was it's nothing, because cancer doesn't hurt in the early stages, so ignore it, and maybe it'll go away. It didn't Still, I didn't tell anyone about it, perhaps subcon-

sciously thinking that discussing the lump would definitely make it real.

For me, cancer was a disease that happened to someone else. There is little cancer in my family's history, and I'd taken all the proper precautions. I'd had an annual checkup and examined my breasts thoroughly each month. When the volunteer rang the doorbell, I gladly gave her a donation.

### REALITY AND DISBEUEF

Unfortunately, doing all the right things doesn't eliminate one's vulnerability to cancer, or make the fact of it any easier to accept The man with heart disease talks about his pacemaker with pride and awe, the diabetic takes his insulin and avoids sweets, proud of his self-discipline, but the victim of cancer is left shattered with disbelief.

I was no different from anyone else. My first hospitalization followed a thorough medical examination, blood tests and a chest X-ray, all of which were negative. However, during the physical exam the surgeon showed extreme concern. He believed that the lump, which was located in a lymph gland, hurt because it was cancer in an advanced stage. He also thought the malignancy had originated in my breast and that a mastectomy would be necessary.

Though I'd thought about cancer, having the doctor actually give credence to my thoughts horrified me. No one is ever prepared to deal with the shocks of life. We either bounce or crumble.

After a biopsy, the node was officially pronounced malignant, and I was given a series of tests to determine the source of the malignancy. A mammogram and upper and lower GI series all proved negative. The surgeon still believed the breast was the culprit and should be removed, but he informed me in no uncertain terms that the primary source might be so small it would never be found, and he might be unable to prove that the malignancy actually came from the breast

## ADDITIONAL ADVICE

Trying to cope with the fect that I had cancer and handling my own rage and frustration while helping my husband, 16-year-old daughter and 13-year-old son deal with the shock they too were living through was difficult enough. Now I had to decide whether to give up my breast I couldn't make that decision without more knowledge, and so I sought additional advice at M.D. Anderson

Hospital in Houston, the cancer medical center of the University of Texas.

At Anderson, I entered a new world. Here, 1,200 cancer patients in all stages of the disease are seen daily on an outpatient basis. I met men and women of every age, race, religion and economic status wasted by the disease, often disfigured and disabled, "suffering from the effects of radiation and chemotherapy, yet fighting and praying for a little more of life. They knew that maybe tomorrow the discovery of a new drug or treatment could prolong their lives. The trick was to make it till tomorrow.

They came to Texas from all over to undergo treatment Smiling and joking, they willingly shared their stories and successes. There was the man who walked slowly because he was so overweight Drinking a thick malted, he said, "You gotta keep eating, then the cancer eats the food, not you." And the woman who readily told me that four years ago she was given a year to live, but thanks to immunotherapy she could proudly display her battle scars.

Always aware of the negative, these people searched out the positive. They had a spirit almost impossible to describe, but I felt it when we were together in the X-ray line or nuclear-therapy waiting room.

My four days of testing again showed nothing. A final medical consultation with a huge group of doctors corroborated my surgeon's opinion that the malignancy must be in the breast since it couldn't be found elsewhere.

With a feeling toward life I'd never known before, I returned home and had the mastectomy. After three days in the pathology lab, the breast finally yielded the primary source of the cancer, the size of a pea buried so deep in the chest wall that I'd have had to be literally turned inside out to have found it There were also three other affected lymph nodes. This gave me a 50-50 chance over the next five years, which improved drastically to 75-25 when I began chemotherapy.

After the surgery I realized how time and preparation had helped me deal with what I had to live with for the rest of my life. How much more fortunate I was than the woman who goes into the hospital for a simple biopsy, and wakes up to find a breast gone.

## THE GIFTS OF TIME

A mastectomy is not a physically debilitating operation, but one you are unlikely to forget Learning to live in a world that idolizes the female breast is not easy. At the beginning one lives with feelings of sexual inadequacy, and the endless questions: Why me? How did this happen? What did I do wrong? Am I less of a woman? Am I cured? Will I live long enough to worry less?

As the wound heals, so does the rage, diminishing the need to ask unanswerable questions that only interfere with living. Time gives each of us the hope that scientists will find more answers and it allows me to share my thoughts to help reduce the fear of cancer so people won't run from their symptoms, but seek care. And perhaps it may make the way a little easier for other victims for me to say that if you must learn to live with cancer, you can.

*Nina Diamond writes a column for The Chattanooga Times.*

# 2

# Moving On

Surgery, generally, means to remove something. If you have lost a breast or had a lump removed, how does this affect your sexual activity or lack thereof? Or does it? What about chemo and the diminution of desire? What about self-esteem? How self-conscious do you feel? Do you hide in the locker room? Do you wear a prosthesis? Did you throw away your lacy bras? When do you tell a new boyfriend? And how? Much time was spent discussing these issues. And, as could be expected, there were "different strokes for different folks" (if you will pardon the allusion.}

Having one side flat, or even both, gave a feeling of incompleteness. Reconstruction took a while to appear on the horizon, and it took a protest march in Boston to secure the right for medical reimbursement for this procedure. Testicular implants had always been reimbursable.

Just deciding whether to undergo the procedure was soul-wrenching. How many more surgeries could we endure? It took several years for this process to improve, and then, many years later some women had to have the prosthesis removed due to medical complications.

Just the fact of having cancer in some way made us feel less; we felt that our bodies had betrayed us.

Our very first educational program in 1978 was about sexuality and self-image. We invited a psychologist from Payne Whitney to speak on the subject of "Sexuality and Breast Cancer." What part does the breast play in our concept of femininity?

When lumpectomies dominated the scene, some of the embarrassment and shame of having only one breast diminished, but the impact of having breast

14

cancer, with all of its ramifications remained With less emphasis on the physical, we could allow our minds to concentrate on our real fears: **Recurrence and Deathl**

We did not forget that having cancer affects the entire family and we started a group for partners and another one for daughters.

One evening when the daughters met in their own group and the mothers met in a separate group parallel to their daughters' group, the mothers heard laughter coming from the other group, and it was clear that the daughters were bonding with one another. Later the groups combined and discussed the issues that arose.

The next day, I received a call from one of the mothers who said that her daughter was a doctor and had not been very emotional or affectionate with her after her diagnosis of cancer. However. after the meeting her daughter drove her home and explained that because she was a medical person she was too aware of all the possibilities that could ensue, and her detachment was a way of protecting herself She kissed her mother good night and told her that she loved her.

It once again affirmed for us the value of peer support and the unlocking of the emotions expressed in a group where each woman was understood and respected.

By this time, many new groups formed, and the women who had the disease facilitated them. We established a more comprehensive training program both for hotline and support group facilitators. These groups were not psychotherapy groups and the main topics were the issues emanating from a cancer diagnosis.

In 1995 an ovarian cancer program was started. It originated with support groups and gradually expanded to include a hotline and participation in national groups dealing with advocacy and research. It is an integral part of SHARE. Ovarian cancer is often very difficult to detect because its symptoms resemble other serious problems. Often, it is not detected until stage three. Much emphasis was placed on educating doctors and women about these symptoms, so that they were not relegated to other non-cancer diseases. This program was initiated by Betty Reiser. It was called the "S.O.S. program(SHARE Ovarian Survivors.)

About this time, in line with our mission of reaching out to under-served communities, several sites were located where African American women could hold their support groups. Warm water aerobics were held at the Harlem Y three times a week … In addition, wellness and education programs were held and emphasis was placed on getting the whole community involved. Rosalind

Donovan, Diane George and Melvina Johnason have been driving forces in this program and Melvina Johnson has facilitated many groups.

Sometimes, we are unable to express our feelings verbally. The pain is so deep within us, that the use of language only exacerbates our feelings.

But there are other methods to help us bring out into the open our experience. One such example is this: One day an art therapist visited SHARE. We all went around in a circle and told the story of our cancer. One woman was unable to speak, and we passed on to the next person.

Then the therapist asked us to draw a picture of our cancer. We all did this and then were asked to talk about it.

Once again, we went around and each person told the others what the picture represented. When it came to the turn of the woman who had been unable to speak, she began to explain her picture with tears in her eyes. The picture was of a woman and a man facing in opposite directions from one another, and the man was walking away from the woman. She explained that the man represented her husband, that he was unable to support her during this trying time, and that she felt completely abandoned by him. This led to a more detailed discussion about her situation and the women drew closer to her and listened carefully and embraced her. In this case, the crayons and paper were the liberating agents that released her from her prison of silence.

The SHARE Hotline was begun just one year after SHARE was founded. In those early days, each volunteer took the responsibility of responding to all Hotline calls for an entire week, on a rotating basis. The telephone was on the floor of someone's closet and the phone bill was paid by a dollar contribution from each member. The average bill was about ten dollars a month. Remember, this was in 1977! Of course, the number of calls received were very few, since SHARE was a small organization at that time.

At the present time, we receive about six hundred calls per month, and we now have over one hundred dedicated volunteers on the Breast Hotline, the Ovarian Hotline and the Latina Hotline. The hotline is available seven days and evenings each week. Calls come from our New York metropolitan area, and also from across the country and occasionally from abroad.

Our hotline is unique is several ways. It is embedded within our peer support organization. Thus, our volunteers and callers have access to all of SHARE'S support, wellness, educational and advocacy programs which meet the array of needs that arise with a cancer diagnosis. All of the Hotline volunteers have been through a training program and continue to attend educational meetings to keep up to date with new medical information. Ongoing training occurs several times a year.

We published a Hotline Newsletter called "The (occasional) Hot Flash."

The Hotline is often the sole support for many women across the nation who are struggling with a new diagnosis or recurrence of ovarian cancer. Many women with ovarian cancer find that there is no ovarian support organization in their geographic area, or even when there is a local support organization, the women may be too ill to attend the meetings in person. The Hotline provides the caller with a life-enhancing connection to women who have traveled the same road and have continued their lives. During the year 2004, 33.6% of its calls came from outside the New York metropolitan area The Hotline is at the heart of SHARE and connects individuals to each and every aspect and program at SHARE such as personal concerns, requests for information regarding resources, support groups and family issues.

Our callers also receive information about clinical trials, symptons, medical and alternative treatments, genetic counseling and many related matters. We do not give medical advice. In December 2005, we received a grant in conjunction with The American Cancer Society to fund a New York State Ovarian Hotline for a year. We also started support group meetings in Queens. We were beginning to expand and word of mouth was a large factor in our popularity.!

By 1983, we introduced wellness programs, which included Yoga, nutrition other exercise programs. Our Yoga program was very popular. And after the meetings, the women often remained to talk about the issues that confronted them.

Four years later, we published our first newsletter for program participants and our contributors, and in 1989, we moved to our new office.

## Yoga at SHARE

### By Roberta Schine

Women come to my SHARE Yoga Class for Women With Breast or Ovarian Cancer hoping to address the question "How can I begin to like, embrace and live in my body after feeling betrayed by it?" They are often in physical and emotional pain. They may be tired, or feeling nauseated if they are in treatment Some are in pain either from recent surgery or from their medication or from metastatic disease. Many come to class after they've finished their treatment but they still feel achy and stiff from having had a somewhat sedentary life for a few months. There is also emotional pain; a sense of loss, anger and fear about an uncertain future. Some women talk about having to deal with ridicule from their doctors and even other people with cancer after making the decision to try alternative treatment. Many experience changes in their body image—weight gain or loss, baldness, the loss of a breast or other part of their body, loss of fertility …

Women also talk about some of the positive changes that may come with a cancer diagnosis. They may feel a sense of pride for having dealt with it. Many have begun to make some positive changes in the way they take care of themselves. Some women develop a new, or deeper, spirituality.

But just about everyone comes to yoga class having experienced profound changes and looking for a way to re-connect with her body.

I try to create a soothing atmosphere where this can begin to happen: I get there before students arrive: I turn off lights and put on soft music, there are mats on the floor, I light candles … Women lie down on mats before the class starts. Class begins with a brief meditation or a poem or a story. Then we do very gentle movements—at first maybe just circling one foot at a time around the ankle or rocking from side to side. I let students know that, if something we do hurts them or doesn't feel right, they need to NOT do it. It doesn't matter if the teacher says it's gentle and everyone around you seems to be enjoying it. I am reminded of what Henry David Thoreau says about bird watching: "If the bird looks different from what the guide-book says it looks like, believe the bird."

Recently, I read an evaluation that one of my students had handed in about the class. In it she wrote, "Roberta gives us permission" She didn't put a period at the end and I wondered what I gave her permission to do. Then one of SHARE'S facilitators suggested that maybe she meant that I give everyone in the class permission to do anything they need to do for themselves. I hope this *is* true in my classes. I provide a structure and give some alternative ways to do things. Sometimes I look around and everyone in the room is doing something different! I once had a student who came to class and lay on the mat without doing one bit of yoga. After the class we sat in a circle and talked and she said she thought the class was terrific! The same thing happened the following week and for several weeks after that. She would bring her stuffed animal, lie down and hug it (it was a little teddy-bear). Once in a while she would stretch out or look around the room and see what the others were doing but that was all. She never did anything I said to do. Then one night, after this had been going on for a few months, she came up to me at the end of class and told me she wouldn't be coming back. She said she had gotten exactly what she needed and thanked me. I said "You're very welcome" and then I added, "But I need to ask you something." She said, "I know, but I really can't talk about that yet Someday I'll tell you." Several months went by and then I received a letter from her. She wrote:" Dear Roberta, I'm so grateful to you for creating a space for me to do nothing. You see, I'm an incest-survivor. And soon after I started to come to terms with that I was diagnosed with cancer. After the incest experience and the cancer experience I had had it with people telling me what I should do with my body. I couldn't even bear to do what a yoga teacher told me to do. I just needed to be in a place where I could focus on my body in my own way. So thank-you for giving me that opportunity."

Chayavida was another wonderful student. She had chosen this name because it means "life" in two languages. Chayavida attended my class for about a year and then she became too ill to come. One day she called me from the hospital and she sounded weak. She said she wasn't doing very well and asked if I would come to the hospital and give her a Yoga class. On the way I realized that she was probably too ill to do yoga so I created a very personal meditation for her that included her favorite colors and places and her grandchildren. When I got to her room I saw that she might even be too sick for that so I asked her if she wanted me to just sit with her. She nodded her head and then seemed to summon all her strength to say "No. Yoga." I couldn't imagine how she was going to do yoga but nevertheless, she had insisted and I was determined to give it a try. So I began the class. She smiled, closed her eyes and lay there without moving a muscle as I led her through arm swings, chest lifts, even balancing poses. Every once in a while I started to feel silly standing in a hospital room giving a yoga class to one person who was just lying there, and I would stop. But then she would immediately open her eyes and look at me in this scolding way—so I would go on. Finally we finished the class, she thanked me and I left. She had taken the whole class—mentally!

There is one other person in the class I want to tell you about—I met her when I first started teaching yoga. She seemed to enjoy the class but at the end she told us she had had a problem with it She said she felt a little guilty about saying this but she wasn't experiencing any of the bad feelings that some of the women in the class talked about. She had lots of energy and felt the class wasn't vigorous enough for her. I was very grateful and realized that to create a truly safe space I would need to address the full range of emotional needs and fitness-levels of my students.

I began practicing yoga when I was diagnosed with breast cancer. I found that it helped me deal with the side effects of treatment and the trauma of the diagnosis. But in those days there seemed to be a war between standard and complementary medicine. I remember the ridicule I felt from my doctor when I told her I was doing yoga. And the Yoga Center I went to put a lot of pressure on me to skip the lumpectomy and just go on a macrobiotic diet. Nowadays we hear about "integrated Medicine" which I think is a much more sensible approach because it says, "Standard medicine has a lot to offer and so does complementary medicine. So let's combine the best from each when we design our health-care strategies," By the way, I'm about to celebrate my 20th cancer-free anniversary!

In 1991, Sally Berg organized the first SHARE Walk. It raised the public awareness about breast cancer and we raised $125,000 to help support our services. It was thrilling to see all of us walking with signs honoring our members, smiling and hopeful and supportive of this organization. The spirit was contagious and we felt like pioneers. We began to ask ourselves "what does empowerment really mean?" We always talked about this subject, and so we decided to hold Patient Empowerment Committee meetings and discover what we meant by the term.

And so we held a series of monthly meetings where we discussed the need for securing more information about effective treatment and how to communicate more effectively with our doctors. We also wanted our doctors to recognize specific cultural diversity issues and address them. We knew we had to play a central role in all of this and needed to bolster our confidence and understand our rights as patients to in order to have more effective medical encounters.

This ultimately led to meetings with medical students and residents where we shared and described the obstacles and challenges in having cancer. They in turn discussed with us the reality of their experiences and some very difficult communication issues they encounter such as breaking bad news. These meetings were ongoing and we exchanged ideas. We expressed the fact that we often felt we were not given enough time to speak, or that we did not understand the explanations (too much "medicalese"). Sometimes we did not have enough time to digest very difficult news i.e. the diagnosis of cancer, or the fact that treatment is no longer working.

We also analyzed our own behavior as patients, such as sometimes not coming prepared with our own priority questions, or not relating pertinent medical facts, or not asking for more medical information and more detailed explanations. The power of hierarchy in medicine often intimidated us, and it took many years for patients to have input into their treatment, to do research and to get second opinions. The various support groups gave us courage and confidence to participate in our own health care. Also, the political climate was changing. The internet and the feminist movement and the strong desire on the part of some doctors to provide a more patient-centered approach, improve communication and in general create a more humanistic relationship led to some changes. The American Academy on Communication in Healthcare helped to pioneer these efforts. Medical schools are now including in their curricula courses on "Relationship Centered Care."

One of the outstanding features of SHARE has been the use of peer support groups for our support groups and our hotline.

Women who have been diagnosed with breast or ovarian cancer facilitate the groups and speak to the callers on the hotline.

This dimension of experience adds credibility and empathy and a level of understanding. SHARE'S use of this model has helped to make us a distinctive presence in the self-help community. Why, you might ask, do we focus so much on experience? Can it make us too subjective? The group is subjective and that is its value. Each person *is* unique and reacts differently to situations they share in common.

That kind of understanding, which is vastly different from the intellectual understanding of something, provides a layer of emotional consciousness, a depth of understanding. We do not underestimate the necessity of cerebral understanding, after all, where would we be without modern medical technology? But at SHARE, we the survivors who have gone through the cancer experience are able to share our feelings, reactions, and coping mechanisms from a visceral understanding of cancer's impact on us personally.

Facing the possibility of death means losing your feelings of invulnerability. It is much like losing the innocence of childhood. We need to feel in control again, even if we know that having control is an illusion in the grand scheme of things. We need to feel that we can take charge of our own bodies, be informed medical consumers, and participate fully in decisions regarding our health. An uninformed choice is not a real choice.

With this in mind, we decided to hold monthly meetings discussing what "empowerment" really means. We discussed how to better communicate with our doctors, to write down our questions before each visit, and to not be afraid to ask them our questions once we were there. We also aimed at becoming better informed about our illness and to change doctors if we were not getting the care or comfort we wanted. We also discussed some cultural differences among Latina and African-American women and how this impacted on the care and treatment we received.

When we dialogue with medical students and residents, we can convey to them what it means to have cancer and how the disease has changed our lives and the lives of our families. We allow them to look inside us and we hope that this vision helps them to see us as total human beings, not a disease entity, and enables them to treat their patients with greater understanding, empathy and a broader view. Since, we are not their patients, there is a more honest and uninhibited interaction. One cannot underestimate the importance of the trust a patient needs to feel towards a doctor in order to make this experience more positive. When that trust is there, there are fewer malpractice suits, more medical compliance and more satisfaction for the doctor. This trust can help to recapture the altruistic reasons the doctor chose the medical profession originally.

In many of the early sessions, we gave examples of insensitive communication on the part of doctors and the anger the doctors aroused in us. As the meetings progressed, we began to consider our part in this duet and what we could do to improve it.

Later, when we met with medical students and residents from NYU and engaged in dialogue with them, we began to understand some of the frustrations and tribulations they experience and we began to look at them as human beings, not gods, as we had done in the past. In learning of others' experiences with doctors, the positive as well as the negative, we began to feel less isolated and more in control. The doctors also learned first-hand what it really feels like to have cancer, from women who spoke from the heart and were not their patients where there might have been some inhibition in frankly expressing themselves.

The support we received from SHARE support groups gave us courage and confidence to participate in our own health care. Also, the political climate was changing and patients were taking a more active stand in participating in a more egalitarian relationship with their doctors.

## Peeling off the Layers

Human beings consist of many parts. Patients often ignore the human part of doctors and doctors often ignore the human part of patients. By choosing to ignore these parts we have denied ourselves the possibility of having a more trusting and fulfilling relationship.

Dr. Tom Ferguson, who spent his life as a physician persuading patients to take control over their own health care and to utilize the Internet in order to accomplish this, once said, "When the doctors get off their pedestals, patients will get off their knees." The converse is also true.

In the year 2,000 we launched partnerships with Bellevue and St. Luke's Hospital in New York City. SHARE Navigators worked in the clinics with the doctors, acting as bridges for the patients to better deal with the hospital bureaucracy, and provide emotional support to help shepherd patients through the hospital system, particularly, the Latina women who did not have fluency in the English language. Our Latina program at SHARE also started support groups for Latina women at St. Vincent's Hospital.

SHARE women have participated in classes of first year medical students directly with the preceptor, and have discussed topics such as "Breaking Bad News". They have observed the role-playing of the students and have also answered the questions posed by the students who valued their experience as patients.

## THE WHITE HOUSE

November 2, 1987

Dear Ms. Miller:

Thank you for your kind message. By sharing your own experience, you have given me strength and encouragement. My husband and I are very grateful for your thoughtfulness and concern.

With our deep appreciation,

Sincerely,

*Nancy Reagan*

Ms. Lee Miller
President
SHARE
6th Floor
817 Broadway at 12th Street
New York, New York 10003

# 3

# Living with Uncertainty

Facing reality can enhance the good times, change your perspective and establish your priorities. You become able to ask questions like, "If not now, when?" We have learned the difference between enlightened self-interest and selfishness. We need to feel we can take charge of our own bodies, be informed medical consumers, and participate fully in decisions regarding our health. An uninformed choice is not a real choice.

We need to feel in control again, even if we know it is an illusion in the grand scheme of things.

Whatever program we have engaged in, whether support groups, education, or advocacy, we derive strength from the knowledge gained by all of us and the commonality of the experience that binds us and validates us. We are not alone and our unity helps us live with this uncertainty.

Each person who has been part of SHARE has left an indelible stamp on us. One such woman was Carol.

The first time I met Carol, she came to volunteer at SHARE after a diagnosis of breast cancer. She began to work with me in the library, and in particular to help organize the books that had been purchased after my husband Ed's death in 1995. The books were purchased from donations received in his memory, and as such, were particularly meaningful to me. From the beginning, she handled all of the books very tenderly, understanding the feelings I had about them. She was very friendly, upbeat and attractive, with eyes that made her resemble Betty Boop!

There had been a delay in her diagnosis, and treatment hadn't started as early as it might have causing her much sadness and some anger.

As we labeled books, sitting at the small round table, we talked of our lives, our cancer and the impact it had made on our lives. She was very involved in her family, her husband, two daughters and a son and their spouses.

She was also very kind. One cold winter day, a homeless man was on the street shivering with cold, and she removed her heavy winter sweater and gave it to him.

As time passed, she became more and more an integral part of SHARE and looked forward to her time spent at our office.

Slowly, her disease started spreading, and she underwent chemo-therapy. One day one of the faxes from her doctor. arrived at our office, indicating that the last test had shown a spread of the cancer. She was very depressed and could hardly speak ... Several of her closest friends sat in the library with her, and we tried to show our concern and love. We hugged her; let her know that we were there for her. Nothing seemed to work. Finally, in desperation, I said, "there is only one thing to do." I ran downstairs and brought up many chocolate bars, and announced to the Staff that chocolate was being served in the "main dining room" (better known as the conference room.)

We all began to laugh, and Carol ate her share of chocolate and actually became cheerful ... I have a feeling there is a moral there, but not everyone shares my love for chocolate.

One day, we were scheduled to meet some residents from NYU Hospital. Several of the SHARE members were to be part of a dialogue with them. We were to discuss our reactions to cancer, our feelings about it, and changes in our lives while living with the disease. Also, we were to tell about some experiences with our doctors including communication (good and bad on both our parts). This was the first time we had done this, and Carol was particularly nervous. We had a small "rehearsal" before the meeting to determine our agenda. Carol had written down her thoughts on the ride into the city because she was fearful that she would not be able to convey her ideas in a spontaneous manner.

We listened to what she had written, and then I suggested that she tear the paper up and just speak from the heart. Which is exactly what happened. The residents sat up and listened attentively, and one of the young men had tears in his eyes when she said that she was buying her Christmas gifts now, because she did not know if she would be around then. After the meeting, he was embarrassed by his tears and Carol knelt down in front of him and said, "Don't be embarrassed; your tears are wonderful and you will be a great "doctor." That's who Carol was ... warm, compassionate and able to reach others without self-pity. She spoke straight from her heart, with respect and caring for those she reached.

She was asked to speak to the first year medical class at NYU. One hundred and sixty students filled the auditorium. The subject was "A Therapeutic Interview" and Dr. Adina Kalet was to interview a metastatic patient. However, it soon became apparent that Carol had a great deal to contribute, and to Dr. Kalet's credit, she permitted Carol to just speak. Carol told how having cancer had changed her life. She spoke of the impact on her family, and her search for more effective treatments including alternative therapies. The students sat spellbound and after the session crowded around her and thanked her for sharing her thoughts and experiences.

The next year she spoke to the new class and this time she had a cell phone with her. She said, "if it rings, I shall run off this stage, because my daughter Susan is about to have a baby. " Well, she did not have to leave the stage, but after the baby was born she sent a picture of her new granddaughter to the class. She was so grateful for having lived to see and love this child. She actually managed to spend the first year with her. She also purchased a new house during the course of her illness because she was determined to live her life to the fullest ... and that she did and she enriched us all with her courage, determination and spirit.

We are accustomed to the idea that when someone we love dies, we enter into a process called bereavement Grief is the emotional reaction we experience regarding this loss.

When we are diagnosed with cancer, do we undergo similar feelings? The answer is decidedly YES!

While death has been an abstraction to us, something that would occur in the future, this diagnosis now makes it real and wipes away the veil that formerly surrounded it. We now know, viscerally that we CAN die and might do so soon. After the shock of the initial diagnosis has worn off and we become somewhat accustomed to the idea, we begin to concentrate on treatment and how to conquer this disease. We also become aware of the secondary losses such as not being able to function in the way we did formerly. If we are undergoing chemo or radiation, we probably will experience side-effects that incapacitate us as least for awhile. We now feel different from our friends and the non-cancer population. We are set apart and we need time to mourn our losses so that we can get through them and go on with our lives. Many of our relationships change, and we now take comfort in the sharing and trust in our support group where others nod their heads in affirmation as we speak. Some of our relationships become closer and we begin to evaluate everything in our lives using different criteria. For example: Am I living my life the way that I now choose? Am I making closer relationships, those that fit my new self? What plans do I wish to carry out? If not now, when?

It takes time to reach these understandings, but in the meantime, we must live with the pain that has accompanied this disease. If we bury it, it will go somewhere else, and affect us negatively. We can only get past it, if we go through it.

SHARE has helped us do that, and the passage of time diminishes the rawness of the emotions.

Everyone's life contains loss and the way we handle it can open up doors to a better life.

Ten years ago, we began forming bereavement groups for those whose family or friends had died of breast or ovarian cancer. We also held an annual Memorial Ceremony honoring those we wished to remember. Poetry and music and a candle-lighting ceremony gave us the opportunity to join together and remember. After the program, we shared some light refreshments, wrote some messages in our "Memory Book" and turned to each other for conversation and comfort.

### BY JENNIFER NEW

# In the name of

LOVE

EXTRAORDINARY OUTPOURINGS OF

DEVOTION IN VERY SPECIAL

RELATIONSHIPS

If you have your eyes set on romance this spring, you might consider whether you're looking in the right direction. Is that special someone the person who will be there for you in a crisis? You might fantasize about candlelight dinners and walks on the beach, but who will still bring you roses when the cards are down? It may not be who you imagined.

Having the love of a special person can be a tremendous comfort for someone dealing with cancer, as the following four relationships illustrate. That love may come from someone who was there all along, or from a wholly new and unexpected source. A woman may meet her true love in the midst of chemotherapy, or remember after treatment that love is a priority. Two of the women profiled here were left by their partners following their diagnoses. But in the end, they all found love, though it sometimes came from surprising places.

Despite her family's close-knit nature, Gloria Heyison could not have foreseen the tremendous love her youngest son would show her as he devoted himself to projects in her honor. Jacqueline Diaz's infant son surprised her, too; one of the tests prior to his birth alerted Diaz to ovarian cancer and, she believes, saved her life. Tara McParland, after discovering she had Stage IV breast cancer when she was just 30 years old, met her life partner and lived twice as long as anyone expected. And Dani Grady learned to take a risk by counting on someone other than herself. Falling in love, she says, was her way of "participating in the world again, of being open to the whole experience of life."

"**Do you know about a small cyst on your left ovary?**" the technician asked Jacqueline Diaz during a routine prenatal ultrasound. Diaz said "no," and then forgot about it as she reveled at the good news: She was carrying a healthy baby boy! At 30 years old, she and her husband already had a daughter and had hoped for a boy. She was "flying" with happiness, she says.

When she walked downstairs to her gynecologist's office, however, she was quickly alarmed. Waiting in the hallway were her doctor and several nurses. They were intensely concerned about the cyst and almost immediately advised Diaz to terminate her 25-week pregnancy in order to take care of her own health and the well-being of her other child. Several days later, a CA-125 test was performed. The blood test, used to screen for ovarian cancer and monitor treatment, should have been a bit above the normal range of 30 to 35 as a result of the pregnancy, but it came back at 2,700.

Of the surgery she underwent to remove the tumor and her ovary less than a week after the ultrasound, Diaz recalls, "It was very grim." If she had gone into labor during the procedure, the baby would have had little chance of survival.

Although he made it through the surgery with flying colors, the doctors remained concerned about her decision to carry the child to term, especially when biopsy results indicated Stage I ovarian cancer.

Diaz held firm. Despite her and her husband's Catholic roots, she says that her decision wasn't about religion; in fact, her doctor even offered to have the Cardinal absolve her. "I could feel the baby kicking inside of me. I already loved him as much as my daughter, and I felt he'd saved my life," she said referring to the early detection from the ultrasound.

She gave birth to baby Joseph on October 7, 1998 and began chemotherapy three weeks later. The family moved in with Diaz's parents so that her mother could take care of the children. There was little that Diaz and her husband—who underwent surgery for a collapsed lung on the same day as Diaz's C-section—could do for children during that time except watch them grow. Still, the children's mere presence helped rouse her from her own sadness and physical pain. "If it wasn't for those kids," she says now without the slightest doubt in her voice, "I wouldn't have gotten through it."

After a brief return to her job in marketing, Diaz spent four years as a full-time mom, calling it the best decision she's ever made. In order to educate and empower other women with cancer, she began working part-time last year for the New York City-based organization SHARE: Self-help for women with breast or ovarian cancer, an organization that played an integral role in her recovery and positive outlook. As the coordinator of the group's ovarian cancer hotline, she shares her story with others. "I'm one of the lucky ones," she tells callers. "I make that very clear. Three years ago I was down in the dumps, and now my life has turned around. Each day is precious, and I'm grateful to share it with my loved ones."

**SHARE'S ovarian hotline can be reached at 212-719-0364 or toll-free at—866-891-2392**

**From Mamm Magazine April,2002**

# 4

# Integration and Absorption

Do we ever get accustomed to the idea of being a person with cancer? Whether we view this as a past or present idea the gravity sticks with us like glue.

How do we live our lives and include this understanding into our psyche? Does the platitude "time heals everything" really work?

We do know that with the passage of time, the wound is less raw; the thoughts previously devoted to this disease diminish if we have not incurred a new or further invasion of it. However, every checkup, every symptom (although seemingly unrelated) re-invokes the fear and the memory. Are we able to pursue the details of our lives without once thinking about cancer?

If the years pass and we remain "stable" (that beautiful word!) other experiences and activities take precedence. Oh, how wonderful it was when I had the flu, and could put that worry in its proper place. Does the cancer we had become part of us, influencing us and changing us without even the conscious realization that it does? Do we take in this addition automatically and accept it as an integral part of ourselves?

Our meetings continued, and when one of our members became metastatic, the fear in each of us multiplied.

One of our members, Patrice discussed the side-effects she experienced from chemotherapy. We understood that each individual is unique and may react to this "poison/medicine" injected into our systems in different ways.

Patrice had a lumpectomy to remove a malignant tumor. This was followed by chemotherapy and radiation and then tamoxifen for two years. Her prognosis was excellent.

However, two years later, she had a recurrence and there was metastases in her liver, lymph nodes and abdomen. She had chemo for four years consisting of taxol; she also took herceptin. In the last year she has only taken herceptin, and has been told she is cancer-free. Also, the various drugs administered caused variations in reaction.

I decided to relate Partrice's experience here because it seems fairly universal. One of her primary concerns was the loss of libido, and fatigue. She felt less desirable on a physical level, and actually said she felt "ugly." The loss of all body hair and the discomfort of her wig contributed to this image of herself. She gave up her job and put all of her energy into treatment and learning more about her disease. This inability to be her "old self" resulted in a tremendous loss of self-esteem. She also wished to reassure her partner that it was not his fault.

When she removed her wig at home, it was always a reminder of her condition. At the same time, she dreaded ending chemo, because at least with it she felt she was actively fighting her disease. The metaport she wears is also a vivid reminder of the treatment she took every week for four and a half years. Her husband volunteered to shave his head, but she refused his kind offer.

She suffers from neuropathy in her hands and feet, and her finger nails have dropped off.

After her chemo ended, she gradually resumed her life, and her sexual life resumed even though she requires a much longer period of stimulation.

The doctors have assured her that she is now cancer-free, although she will be on this special medication for the rest of her life.

Several years after Patrice's experience, the need arose for women with metastatic cancer to have their own group. A psycho-therapist and cancer survivor herself, Roberta Huffnagel initiated this group so that the women could talk to each other about the effects this advanced form of cancer had on their lives. Today, metastatic women are realizing that they need to speak for themselves, and are making themselves more visible in the advocacy community. So the question remains,"Can we absorb and integrate this cancer experience into our lives and accept it as an integral part of our lives?"

I believe that we can and the absorption of this experience adds a dimension to our lives both positive and negative in that the pain and fear have given rise to re-examining our priorities and hopefully intensified our ability to love and appreciate the joy of life.

# 5

# Cancer is International

About thirty years ago, Americans started their fight against breast cancer from a low level of awareness. Women began to be outspoken about this disease and conquered their feelings of embarrassment. They took it "out of the closet" and brought the medical, social and emotional issues to the forefront.

Through the efforts of Marcia Presky, a member of SHARE and associated with The American Jewish Joint Distribution Committee a small task force of women visited Israel. They also visited Poland, Ukraine and the Czech Republic beginning in 1995 ... In general, we sought to share our experiences with the disease and encourage women to take a more active part in the prevention, detection and treatment of breast cancer. We felt they needed to develop a more egalitarian relationship with their physicians, and that there should be a more empathic attitude on the part of the doctors. These women were encouraged to develop support groups, to lobby for new laws protecting health, to engage in fund-raising in order to enhance the quality and availability of essential equipment and supplies, and to secure patient education materials for wide distribution.

Visits by the Americans were made to hospitals, to existing cancer organizations, and to non-governmental organizations active in women's health.

It was very exciting to visit a country and meet the women who had breast cancer. We knew that we were more open in our discussions about the disease, and less modest and able to more freely verbalize our feelings about the disease and to discuss it with others.

Although, we observed some differences in their feelings about privacy and relationships with their partners, the desire to help others and conquer this disease was universal.

In each country warm ties were established between the American women and the foreign women lasting until the present.

We learned that the universality of the effects of this disease, the concerns, and the similarities were far greater than the differences among us. Not only were we teachers, but students as well, learning from each other and uniting in our desire to conquer this disease and to share our knowledge and support with others. In that way, we were helped ourselves. We had already learned that lesson from SHARE.

We continued to keep abreast of the new programs these women had inaugurated and to feel a sense of pride in our association with them.

## Se Habla Espanol?

By 1992, we had an increasing number of Latina members. Some of them spoke English, some Spanish and some were bi-lingual. It became apparent that conducting support groups in Spanish made many of the members feel more comfortable and we were able to convey medical information in a more informative and understandable manner.

Alexandria Colon, who had been trained as a facilitator and was a breast cancer survivor started the first group.

It was a feeling of great relief for the women to be able to express themselves in their native tongue, and to have the various issues that arose be understood in the context of their cultural values. They not only provided support to each other within the group, but outside the group as well. They accompanied one another to treatment, visited their families and allowed family members to attend the group, including children. When a woman was hospitalized they visited her and often prepared food for the family. One woman restored wigs and prostheses and made them available to others. There is generally food served at the meetings, which differs from practices in the other groups. There are many awards given to the women in recognition of services rendered. There is an atmosphere of acknowledgement and praise for all.

As an example of the needs addressed by the program, one of the women knew that she was dying. The facilitator, Alex chose not to let her die alone, since all of her relatives lived outside of the United States. When this woman was in a hospice setting, Alex stayed with her and held her hand as she lay dying, Later, the women contributed money so that the woman's closest relative could be here for the funeral.

The group also has many educational discussions. Doctors, nurses and nutritionists have spoken on topics such as lymphedema, metastatic disease, post-mastectomy care, meditation, relaxation, wellness programs, aroma therapy and Reiiki (wellness circle with hands-on healing). A hotline in Spanish was introduced and many calls are received Many materials have been translated into Spanish, such as suggestions for more effective patient-doctor communication.

We know that cancer is color-blind and SHARE has reached out to many under-served communities, ethnically diverse groups and to every woman wishing to avail herself of our services without charge.

In the year 2000, a Peer Navigation Project was started in which a SHARE member was stationed at a clinic to help the patient navigate the complexities of the medical system, and help explain medical procedures and treatment and offer support.

Perhaps the test way to describe Latina SHARE is with the following story, from the daughter of one of the women who was very introverted and depressed after her diagnosis of breast cancer. After joining a group, which had appeal because the meeting was conducted in Spanish and thus enabled the mother to have a feeling of belonging, the mother was invited to participate in a meeting at the National Breast Cancer Coalition held in Washington, DC. This was an advocacy training conference. The daughter, said "It was like the cracking of a shell when my mother banged her fist on a Congressman's table."

The following letter, which her daughter wrote to SHARE, captures the meaning that Latina SHARE had for her mother:

*"What comes to mind when I think of SHARE? Their pursuit of eliminating any and all barriers that get in the way of their participants' healing process. Therefore, it should come as no surprise that they formed Latina SHARE. A complementary unit that caters to the needs of women who take great comfort in garnering their support from peers in their native Spanish tongue. This endeavor is just one of the many progressive strides that SHARE makes, and all in the effort to achieve the very best standards of care for the women who seek their assistance.*

*My mother was one of those women ... and to say that Latina SHARE transformed my mother's life is truly an understatement. No words can encapsulate the impact that Latina SHARE has made in her life. It revolutionized the way she thinks about cancer. It revolutionized the way she thinks about health care. And, most importantly, it revolutionized the way she thinks about herself and her ability to claim her strength back after such a debilitating experience. No longer was cancer considered a death sentence. She came to learn of women in her own support group who had survived this monstrosity of a disease and live to tell about it. Latina SHARE is an invaluable resource for women like my mother who migrated here from afar to create a new life, amidst the challenges of being a foreigner. Latina SHARE saw to it that in her journey to regain her health, it minimized any further challenges. It also taught her how to be an advocate for herself in the face of all modern medicine's complexity.*

*They helped her reclaim her spirit back ... and for that I am eternally grateful."*

*Vanessa*

## Some Additional Facts: Statistics

### Hispanics/Latinas

Hispanic/Latina women show lower breast cancer screening rates that non-Hispanic/Latina White women and tend to seek and attain health care services less frequently than other ethnic groups. However, breast cancer is the most commonly diagnosed cancer among Hispanic/Latina women; an estimated 14,300 Hispanics/Latinas are expected to be diagnosed in 2006. An estimated 1,740 deaths from breast cancer are expected to occur among Hispanic/Latinas in 2006. Studies also show that even though Hispanic/Latina women have lower breast cancer rates, they are 20% more likely to die from the disease. This contradiction is due to the fact that Hispanic/Latina women are less likely to participate in mammography screening and more likely to be diagnosed at later stages of breast cancer. Studies consistently show that low income, low educational attainment, lack of health insurance, inability to speak English, lack of awareness of breast cancer risks and screening methods, acculturation level and lack of physician referral play important roles in the lower rates of screening utilization by Hispanic/Latina women.

Source: http://www.komen.org/intradoc-cgi/idc_cgi_isapi.dil?
IdcService=SS_GET_PAGE&ssDOCNAME=BreastFacts
Statistics#hispanicslatinas

Breast cancer is the most commonly diagnosed cancer and the leading cause of cancer death among Hispanic American/Latina women. Hispanic whites are more likely to be diagnosed with tumors that are more advanced than are non-Hispanic whites and Asian/Pacific Islanders. Women of Mexican, South and Central American and Puerto Rican descent are 20% to 260% more likely to be diagnosed with late-stage breast cancer when compared to non-Hispanic women. When looking at breast cancer treatment, Puerto Rican women fare the worst, as they are 50% more likely to receive poor, inappropriate treatment. And Mexican women have 30% poorer survival rates when compared to non-Hispanic whites.

Source: USHHS National Women's Health Information Center
http//www.4woman.gov/minority/hispanicainerican/bc.cfm

We need specific health statistics of the various subsets of Latina/Hispanic target groups within the U.S.A.

# 6

# Bonnie's Story

In 1995, the need arose for us to start an Ovarian Program. We began with a small group of ovarian cancer survivors and started a support group. Women are often at high risk because the diagnosis often does not occur until well into the disease. The symptoms can be indicative of many other things and because of this, we have been very involved in creating awareness about early detection through education and outreach to the medical community and general public.

Perhaps a more personal picture of this program can be understood through the words of one of our young survivors, Bonnie.

October 1988—I was Eighteen.

"I was the precarious age of eighteen. I had just recently graduated from high-school and was away at college for my first semester of dorm/campus university life. My newfound freedom of living without parents, curfews or limits was suiting me well. It was what I had been anticipating. I was a theater major and spreading my wings fully for the first time, re-creating myself on my own.

At the first of October, I found myself with the dilemma of a very sore throat. I debated whether or not to just sleep it off, or go check it out. My new friend Lori, who also had a sore throat, rationalized that we should go to the clinic and get some medicine, since we were both insured with campus health care coverage. Perhaps it was just the shove I needed. We journeyed cross-campus through the quad, over to the University clinic. I remember the chilly, achy walk.

After what seemed like hours, I was finally seen by the doctor. I immediately made reference to the round belly that I had been accumulating. I had attributed it to very poor eating, a lot of late nights and binge eating, pizza galore and chocolate. Not to mention plenty of beer drinking ... for the first time ever. When I saw his reaction, I think my words were, "oh, I'm getting fat."

Obviously, the doctor was concerned because he asked if I could be pregnant, asked about my periods, and whether or not I had been to an OB/GYN. I laughed and told him that I was definitely not pregnant since I was a virgin, had not been to an OB/GYN, and that my periods were always irregular. I heard that happened to a lot of girls.

The doctor listened to me attentively, but then took his time, looked me in the eye and said, "I really need you to promise me that before you leave this office you will go see the OB/GYN.to whom I shall refer you. There was a very concerned tone in his voice.

The office was at the end of the hall. A nice nurse was there with me and held my hand because I was terrified of my first pelvic exam. Needless, to say, the exam was quite painful Just as I expected, the doctor and I did not communicate very well He was a middle-aged Chinese man and all I remember him exclaiming was the word "tumor." This was after I had to convince everyone that I was not pregnant. All I really remember him saying was that I should get some tests and see my family OB/GYN.

I barely remember leaving his office. During the walk back across campus, I felt numb and my eyes welled with hot tears.

Lori and I decided to go back to the theater building because that is where I wanted to go. I saw my friend Don, and I felt safe pouring out the whole story to him. I literally cried on his shoulder, though I don't remember what I said.

My friends told me to call my parents but I just could not do it. I think I was terrified about their reaction. I felt somehow responsible and I did not wish to leave. I decided to call my older sister, Donnette and she could help me figure out what to do. I called my sister from a pay phone in the building. I felt very comfortable telling her what had just happened. She was immediately and intensely concerned and she said she would drive down to see me that night.

What a blur the next few hours were! I must have gone back to my dorm and taken a nap and spoke to my roommates. Having sobbed with Don and talked to my sister, I was already feeling calmer. I felt like I had already shared some of the burden of this whole thing. I felt less alone. But, I would soon come to realize how alone you really feel when your own mortality is introduced to you for the first time.

My sister arrived quite late and I insisted that we go out with my buddies to the quad theater, then to a late night theater party and hang out and drink and smoke till the wee hours. My sister was appalled that I refused to talk about my situation that evening and that I could indulge in a full eve of festivities. I remember having a really good time that night and laughing my ass off. It was as if I were going off to war. I knew it deep inside. The party would be over for me now. The freedom gone. I was going to have to leave school. I wasn't exactly thinking this that evening, but now I know why I was so reckless that night. It was my send-off party to myself.

I really did not want to get the ball rolling, but my sister made me sit down with her the next day and call our parents. I do not really remember the phone call. I am sure I was aloof and distant because that was my way of keeping my fear factor low. My dad was able to get me to agree to ride home with him the next day, Sunday, so that I could see Dr. Baron-Kuhn, the OB/GYN at home, and have tests. I was obsessed with not losing out on the whole semester, and I wanted to miss no more than a week of school. My dad was good at minimizing the situation for me, and had me half-convinced that this should be an in-and-out thing and I would still be able to finish the semester. It was what we were all hoping for anyway.

I remember that autumn three hour ride back to Chicago. We spoke of other things. I tried to just day-dream out the window. The sky was beautiful.

I saw Dr. Baron-Kuhn that Monday. She was so gentle and kind and sweet, and so careful as she examined me. It did not seem so painful She looked me in the eye with her hands on my knees and said "okay kid, honest, no sex?" She made me crack a smile and I said "nope, no sex. "She had a similar prognosis as the other GYN but she ordered many tests to be taken at the hospital.

The mass in my abdomen was quite big, and the ultrasound showed complexities. An exploratory surgery was quickly scheduled. After getting some more test results, my mom and I were returning to the house from a giddy shopping spree for hospital slippers, etc. when my sister came out of the house with a very disturbed look on her face. She told us that the doctor had just called and wanted to move the surgery up to tomorrow. She also wanted us to come right to her office after we returned home. Right then and there was a defining moment … I fell to my knees in the front yard, weeping, saying "this can't be good. Why did she call if it's not bad?" I just cried and cried with my parents as they hugged me and they probably cried too. Then we pulled ourselves together to go see Dr. Baron-Kuhn.

We met and sat with her in her consultation office. It was a very handsome room. My mom and my dad and me. Just like how I started out.

It was a beautiful sunny day. I do not remember the medical jargon, but I remember Dr. Baron-Kuhn behind her own choking tears telling us that there was a fifty/fifty chance that this was cancer and there were some strong concerns that came from my test results, which warranted this visit She was moving surgery to the next day, and she was bringing in an expert GYN/ONC to perform the surgery with her. I will never forget Dr. Baron-Kuhn being so teary-eyed and heartfelt during this conversation. She was full of deep compassion and feeling and was right there with us. We were a team and she became our angelic hope. We hoped the doctor could save me. We were all fighting back tears. There were important arrangements and tests that had to be done.

After we left the office, or maybe I even fled the office, I remember bursting into tears outside the office and soaking my dad's shirt. I asked him if I was going to die like Nanna did. He said NO! of course not. He was crying too. It was scary. I realized no one could make this situation safe and assured.

I proceeded to be tested and x-rayed from head to toe, and had to fill out a ton of pre-surgery paperwork. I didn't mind the tests, CT scans with injections (MRI'S and PET scans were not even invented yet!) The tests kept me busy, they were strange, lonely and distracting and yet gave me time to think or just doze off. The only thing that made me feel nervous was having to sign my life away to anesthesiology! The enema the night before the surgery was a horror but the drugs from the IV right before the surgery that day were quite relaxing. The scheduling of the surgery was of course, running behind, and I remember how relaxed I was from the IV and trying to calm down my poor pacing parents. My worst concern (hear the voice of the vain eighteen year old) was that there was a small chance that my bladder might be involved and I would need a colostomy and I would need it in order to relieve myself. That I could not accept. I remember knowing that I could handle any result except that.

The surgery was well over six hours, and my tormented family waited. I had one or two blood transfusions. Somewhere, around the three hour mark, the doctor came out and told my parents that it was a malignant tumor and it had spread. They were trying to remove all of the diseased area. They were meticulously sure to remove everything that had spread, and it really had spread. The result was Ovarian Cancer Stage IIIC-Dysgerminoma/Carcinoma and they had performed a hysterectomy and one ovary was left. There was a ten inch scar right down my belly.

I had a hysterectomy with one ovary left, slept through recovery and one day after that. I remember waking up and someone saying "Bonnie, this was cancer" and I mumbled "Is my bladder ok? "Do 1 need the bag?" And they said that it was just fine, but I did have cancer. Then, I said "As long as the bladder is ok, well that's ok then." Then, I think I slept for two days.

I believe I had a hospital stay of almost ten days Lots of flowers, the stitches hurt, especially when my dad or TV made me laugh. Lots of TV which was a rarity in my house. Lots of visitors and friends from high school, and family. Since I was always an over-extended, too busy and fatigued person, I remember subtly enjoying the downtime. Even if I wanted to, I couldn't be busy. I just had to relax. To this day, I am still forced to relax by ill health. I thought, prayed and talked to God and remembered my pact that I could handle anything except wearing a bag. This can't be it, I said. Uh-uh, no way. This is not it; this *is* not the end for me. This was a quick epiphany, but I rode it all the way home to remission. And the important thing is, I did believe this in my heart. And I felt it was partly my decision (whether I died or not) and I could choose to believe this (give-up or not.)Well, I escaped the fate of the colostomy bag, so I decided to escape this fate too and not give up. There's too much more, I choose to believe that I am going to get better. I have to!

I was faced with the decision, radiation or chemo. This was frustrating. My oncologist highly recommended localized radiation for thirty rounds with boosts to the upper and lower abdomen. I was toying with chemo because my sister was trying to let me know I could freeze eggs that way from one remaining ovary. I was confused! My parents wanted to just do as my oncologist, Dr. Sweet, would suggest, and also not waste time freezing eggs. I already had a bone-marrow harvest. I almost went the chemo route and once again the doctor looked me in the eye and said "Bonnie, your type of cancer has most successfully been treated by radiation. I am a chemo therapist and I tell you, you don't need to have that poison put into you, don't. But, let me know what you decide" Well, it was just the shove I needed. I went for the radiation as the text book suggested, and counted down thirty days, Monday—Friday that took me right through December.

The days were hazy. I was fatigued and nauseated. I vomited daily. I didn't do too much during that time, Just slept. I forced myself to eat. Watched some TV. I couldn't really read books or write.

After radiation was completed, with the doctor's permission I was able to go back to college (Jan. '89) This was a promise that got me through treatment. I had waited eighteen years for this freedom and then I had to wait three more months. I had made it! Campus is where I needed to be. That got me through.

And I did return, and left in 1989, and then returned to Community College and left again in '93, and returned in '94 and left again.

I coasted through much of my twenties unscathed by the wounds of my disease, and plunged into a daily routine full of fun and excitement. Rarely was I confronted with many of the issues from being ill. And when I was slightly confronted, I redirected myself to some other exciting adventure. I worked hard and played hard. I had put myself in a safe circle. I traveled a lot and went on many spiritual quests through visits to beautiful natural wonders. For a relatively long period of time, I had a close boyfriend and he was very cool about my menopausal side-effects and sexually low libido.

Then, just before my thirtieth birthday, I really felt the enormity of my illness and understood the intense seriousness that was always reflected on the faces of my family and doctors.

That autumn I found myself typically October blue, since that had been the time of my surgery and diagnosis.

My Mom found SHARE on an internet search and recommended that I check out the organization, since I live in Manhattan. I was nervous about getting involved since I was so many years past diagnosis and treatment. I wasn't sure I would fit in (once again!)

It took me almost a year to call. I finally did and for the first time met young women who also had ovarian cancer. The meeting was full of wonderful dynamic, smart and vibrant women. It was a powerful setting, and I became very involved with these support meetings And now, after an interneship with SHARE, I facilitated these monthly meetings as well as work for the SHARE hotline for ovarian cancer calls. I did this twice a week and have received both facilitation and hotline training. My involvement with SHARE has been the very essence of the SHARE motto"experience is our expertise"; peer-led support.

I look forward to having a career in the field of cancer support services. I remember listening to others' dismay as I would share my story, or as loved ones recalled the occurrence. I was just so happy to be alive I just couldn't grasp their sorrow over it yet It hadn't caught up with me and I put it I a safe place emotionally. I was here to live for the moment.

When I was thirty-two I attended a Human Sexuality Class. It was the summer of 2002, fourteen years past my cancer diagnosis. I was interested and fascinated, since I had read many books on the topic to overcome and understand my post-hysterectomy/menopausal female body. I was always dealing with being in a relationship, so I didn't really ignore sex, although I could have.

Anyway, the class was fascinating. However, during the course of it, I found myself just mystified by the fact that I was missing some of the basic female anatomy. I requested my medical records and finally looked them over. I understood how much of me had been removed from my body and I began to understand even more of the side-effects. I was wowed by my survival Phew!! I really was a bit of a walking miracle. I asked my doctors and family questions and I got closer to the reality of having had stage 3-C cancer.

The issue of children and family seemed to hit me around age thirty-three or thirty-four. It comes up involuntarily; when I am hearing a story about someone's pregnancy or baby story. The miracle of pregnancy, even periods sometimes leave me feeling isolated and resentful. I never knew I had these feelings until recently. It *is* as if they came out of nowhere. I guess it is my age (35) and listening to many peers who discuss their biological clocks that have begun to tick. There is a strange feeling for me when I attend baby showers now. I have discussed this with other women at SHARE meetings and we have had some fantastic round table discussions about our similar emotions and reactions.

Another thing that stirs up my resentment is seeing violent parents, or spoiled rich children. Such issues have stirred anger in me about not having the option and my own opportunity to raise a child. Remembering my warm family makes me recall that familiarity that a family really does bring. I never had time to ponder these issues before.

I am glad to have a dog to shower with love and care as well as a wonderful man whom I respect and adore.

The isolated feeling of not bearing children or making a family fades once there is a club of women who have the same issue ... the same loss ... at the same cost. That is SHARE!

That is why support groups are so effective and provide much relief. And to have a facilitator who is a survivor keeps that bond so much tighter.

In conclusion, I am glad I have finally experienced the emotional reactions to my cancer. I have recently been confronting the issues as they come up in their own time. I could never say I wish this hadn't happened to me, because this experience is the basis of who I am today. It's even hard to imagine who I would be if I had not undergone this experience. I am grateful for the chance to survive and hope to live a long time!

I have graduated from Hunter College after many starts and stops along the way. I am now living in Florida and on July 4, 2006, I married the man I adore. And now, I am ready for my future!

# Source: Lifetime Online—Health: Breast Cancer Survivor Profile

**Finding Strength in Strangers**
When Elma Denham was diagnosed with cancer, all she wanted was a stranger to talk to.

by Sara Eckel

When Elma Denham's doctor assured her that the shadow on her mammogram was probably nothing, she believed him. After all, she had no family history of breast cancer, and Denham, then 68, was in perfect health. But after the biopsy, her doctor walked into the recovery room and blurted out that Denham had cancer—then he left. "He was so shocked that he couldn't even talk to me," remembers Denham. "So I was just lying there, absolutely stunned."

As a mother who raised two daughters—and a social worker who assisted young people and their families in New York City—Denham had spent her entire life caring for others She had always been the strong one, the person who provided comfort and answers; but the breast cancer diagnosis left her feeling helpless and confused.

Vowing to never be so blindsided again, Denham immediately began researching her condition, but the jargon-laced medical reports raised more questions than they answered. The doctors weren't much better, rattling off a slew of polysyllabic terms and then dashing out the door before Denham could absorb them all. "I was so befuddled. The doctors didn't make sense," she says.

Even her brother, an oncologist, couldn't clarify things for her. "He told me about a lot of important medical stuff, but not in a way that I needed it explained," says Denham.

Denham didn't know where to turn. None of her friends had had breast cancer, so not one of them could understand her situation. Her daughters, Stacey and Lisa, were supportive: Stacey flew in from Germany, and Lisa spent weekends cooking and visiting Denham at her New York City apartment. But Denham hid her deepest fears from them. "You don't want to burden your family, because they're scared too—but they don't want you to know that," she says.

Finally, Denham's research led her to SHARE, a support group for women with breast or ovarian cancer The first day she went to SHARE's office near Times Square, it was as bustling and crowded as the city outside. Her group was comprised of 11 other newly diagnosed patients, including a lawyer, a stay-at-home mom and a psychologist. "I immediately felt at home," says Denham (pictured with other SHARE members, below), who told the others about her worries for her daughters

—her fears that they would get the disease. Then one woman replied, "Right now we need to talk about you."

"That really helped me," says Denham. "My way of dealing with things is to be helpful to the others. It was very hard for me to ask for help, because I've always been the helper—personally and professionally." For the first time, Denham talked about how she felt: angry, scared and exhausted.

Members gave her practical advice on everything from creams to soothe her radiation burns to strategies for dealing with the amazing vanishing doctors. "It had never occurred to me to bring a tape recorder [ medical appointments], or to bring a friend along to take notes," she says. "But after that, a SHARE volunteer accompanied me to all my radiation treatments. That was wonderful."

At SHARE, Denham found a community, a place where people didn't just sympathize, they truly understood. "You come in with anxiety [because] you have a test [coming up] and they just see it on your face. They say, 'What's going on? When's your appointment? Who are you seeing?' I don't even have to say anything; they just see it."

This kind of empathy can only come from a fellow survivor, says Denham. "Your friends and family want to buck you up, to make you feel good. They think, you're finished with radiation now, so you can get on with your life. But that's not how it is. It is on your shoulders all the time, sure you still go out to the movies and the theater, but it's always there," she says.

That's why Denham's involvement in SHARE didn't end with her treatment. Her support group continued for a year, then she became a volunteer. And in February, 1999, she was hired for a staff position. She was the coordinator of hospital-based programs.

But it was November, 1996, when Denham faced her most difficult role: that of a care giver once again. Her daughter Lisa was diagnosed with breast cancer. "It was much harder, "she says. "I was absolutely terrified all the time." Denham stayed with her daughter in New Jersey during the week, but she says her contact with SHARE crucial during Lisa's illness—and after Lisa's death in February 1998. I don't know how I could have survived that time without SHARE," says Denham. "They would call and say 'we're thinking of you. We are praying for you. You don't have to reply, no obligation, but know that we care.'"

# 7

# "Sharing the Experience"

We all know that cancer affects the patient in a most direct way. But, how about the family, the children, the friends? In SHARE we have all found different venues for coping.

The Children's Group founded by Elma Denham in 1996 dealt with the impact of a parent's cancer on the child ... There were monthly meetings where the children ages (seven to twelve years) met and played games and ate food and talked to one another. Younger and older siblings were always welcome at the meetings. While they did this, their mothers met in another room and spoke and supported each other. The children were free to roam in and out and became accustomed to hearing words like "chemotherapy" "recurrence" and "cancer." They observed the wigs some of the mothers wore and the new hair grown in by others. This gave them a familiarity with the disease and helped them understand that they were not alone. They met for several years and some became teen-agers with leadership roles.

Seven years ago, some youth leaders were trained through Kids Konnected in California. As a result, a teenager who was trained facilitated these meetings at SHARE.

Then, a long weekend at a camp in California was offered to all of the members of the group. The weekend was paid for by the California Kids Konnected Group and we raised the money for the fare so that all of the children could attend They had a wonderful time and learned skills that will be of help to them for the rest of their lives!.

We also have a group for seniors which has met for years. They meet bi-monthly and discuss the concerns they have as "Survivors Growing Older." They are a closely-knit group and have close bonds with each other.

There are those members who wish to put their energies into advocacy. In 1994 the National Breast Cancer Coalition created a crash course in epidemiology and basic science. One year later, the Coalition brought together a group of advocates, scientists and clinicians to design the first Project Lead curriculum. The structure provides breast cancer advocates the tools they need to influence research and public policy, and for members from all over the country to participate actively in the wide range of forums where decisions about breast cancer are made.

Over the last eleven years, Project Lead has held more than forty-four courses four to five times a year. Over eleven hundred people from forty-eight states and forty-one countries have graduated and there is a waiting list for students eager to participate.

## Adrienne's Story

It was a sunny day in July of 1999. I went for my routine mammogram and was very upset and started shaking from fear when the radiologist told me there might be a problem. This was the beginning of a dramatic turning point in my life.

A few weeks later I had a surgical biopsy (a lumpectomy). When the pathology report came back, I was shocked like any other woman would be upon hearing the words "Breast Cancer."

Both my parents had died from cancer, seventeen and eighteen years before. Thus I had a fear of getting cancer, but it was of colon and pancreatic cancer. However, breast cancer was not a conscious concern of mine.

After the shock of being told I had breast cancer wore off, I was very grateful that my cancer was caught early. I was diagnosed with stage one invasive ductal carcinoma. Thirteen lymph nodes were removed but there was no nodal involvement. I received thirty three radiation treatments over a six and a half week period.

After I got the diagnosis, my chiropractor told me about SHARE. I called the SHARE hotline and at a later point in time, I joined a support group for newly diagnosed women with breast cancer. I was relieved to be able to share my fears and concerns with other women who really understood. And now six and a half years later, I still meet with the members of my support group. We have become friends or as some would say, "sisters."

I am a very spiritual person. And in spite of all the grief and sadness I have felt from losing my mother, father, and brother to cancer, and having had cancer myself—I believe that out of bad situations good can come if you let it. I now have more perspective and acceptance of those things I cannot change.

The journey of life is very mysterious. I never could have imagined on that sunny day in July of 1999, that the results of my routine mammogram would have such an impact on my life.

After retiring from teaching in 2000, I wanted to give back to SHARE. Thus, since January of 2001 I have been a volunteer at this wonderful organization. SHARE, you were there for me in my time of need and I will always be grateful. Thank You."

No amount of money could ever give me the satisfaction that I feel when I volunteer at SHARE knowing I am helping other women who have been diagnosed with breast or ovarian cancer. As the adage goes "To Give is to Receive."

# 8

# Some Random Thoughts

How does one cope with cancer? Is it possible to adjust to this deadly disease? Is it just a matter of time that helps us become accustomed to living with the idea that our lives may be prematurely shortened? Or as time goes by, is cancer just a part of our lives, and as we live longer and the days are filled with the details of living do we put the idea on the back burner and gain more confidence? There is always hope, and the possibility of new treatments. In fact, some remarkable strides have already been made.

What have we learned during the hundreds and perhaps thousands of support groups that seem to answer this question? Well, first of all, we learn that we are all different and as unique individuals we react differently. But, are there some universal lessons we have learned? I believe there are.

One of them is the knowledge that we are not alone; support groups affirm this all the time. The support of family and friends contributes to our feelings of well-being in general and supply a protective shield for us. Learning all that we can about the disease helps many, and trust and confidence in the competence of the physician is most important Also, the knowledge that we are in a partnership with our doctors and they are here for us through the good times and bad times. The examples other women set for us in terms of courage and inspiration give us goals we can emulate.

Perhaps we each find our own answer. Although life is uncertain, we have had this affirmed for us. That is the reality of life and our cancer has helped us deal with that reality.

It is a lesson we would rather not have learned this way, but perhaps this knowledge helps us deal with life in general. Anyway, we hope so!

But how does the doctor tell the patient she has cancer? Is there any easy way to do this? How can the patient absorb this horrendous news in one gulp? Do thoughts of death immediately occur to her? Probably.

What do we mean by "candor with hope?" What can the hope be if the prognosis is uncertain? Well, there are new treatments on the horizon addressing the whole spectrum of the disease.

Often, patients ask, "How long will I have to live?" It is a question that cannot be definitively answered ; statistics are only relevant if they apply to you. So then, where is the hope? The hope is that there will be a relationship where, if you desire, (and some patients do not) you will understand in com- prehensible terms what the medication and treatment are expected to do. This includes the possible side-effects and the expected benefits. You will be heard and your input valued. In a sense, this kind of "Relationship-Centered Care" provides the hope one needs to manage this illness and a determination on your part to struggle and live your life to the fullest under the circumstances.

It is our hope that in the future, this type of "relationship-centered care" becomes the norm and that it will not only help the patient cope, but help to satisfy the altruistic reasons for which one entered the medical profession in the first place. It is a "win/win" situation and that kernelof trust and sharing can blossom into HOPE!

## Compensatory Living

Two of the definitions in Merriam-Webster's dictionary for "compensate" are "to neutralize the effect of or "to provide the means of counteracting variation." In this case the "variation" would be the cancer.

So are there any positive outcomes from having breast or ovarian cancer? Is this just a rationalization? Perhaps it is. Nonetheless, can we or do we achieve any compensation in the same way had we not had the disease?

What might these compensations be? From the findings of hundreds of support groups, several responses occur over and over; always with the statement "I would rather not have cancer, but having had it, I can pull out of this experience some positives." They are usually: valuing the importance of each day, not wasting time with non-essentials, treasuring the love and friendship that I have in my life, making decisions I have always wanted to make and have delayed, and expressing my positive feelings to others with much greater frequency than I have in the past. So you might ask "why didn't these learnings occur in pre-cancer days?" Perhaps because in the rush and the details of ordinary life, we are engaged in action and do not often take the time to reflect on our feelings. What we have, we take for granted. We often dwell on the negative aspects of life, the things that go wrong, and do not appreciate what we do have. Anyway, that is how it seems to me. Are we ever the same after the diagnosis? Definitely not! Are we wiser or more empathic? Perhaps, but being part of a support group helps underscore these positives and helps us absorb the pain of this "variation."

## Is Having Breast Cancer a Small Death?

If death constitutes loss, and the need for grieving is a natural concomitant of that loss, are we able to fully absorb the pain, accept the loss and then go on?

What have we lost?

We have lost the belief that we are invulnerable and have control over our lives. Did we have control over the cancer that assailed us? Is the idea that death is inevitable made more real after a diagnosis of cancer? And how does that understanding affect us?

Are we beset by fears, anxiety and a diminished capacity to enjoy life? Is the first thought upon waking up in the morning, "I have cancer?" We begin the difficult journey of understanding that our loss is real. We allow ourselves to experience the pain of grief in all of its forms. There are no shortcuts through the pain.

As Therese Rando has written (with some editing) the three tasks of grief are:

1.  understanding and acknowledging the loss

2.  experiencing the pain reaction to the loss

3.  Moving adaptively into the new life

Even though you feel that you have been irrevocably changed by the cancer, your core remains the same.

We eventually come to a point where we choose to say "yes" to life again. And in this case, with the "little death" you are resurrected into a full human being embodying this experience and moving on. It is interesting to note that the word "embodying" contains the word "dying" within it and the word "body" as well. Perhaps the "little death" has died within the body and life goes on.

# Grief

We are all accustomed to the idea that when someone we love dies, we enter into a process called bereavement. Grief is the emotional reaction we experience regarding this loss.

When we are diagnosed with cancer, do we undergo similar feelings? The answer is decidedly YES!

While death has always been an abstraction to us, something that would occur in the future, this diagnosis now makes it real and wipes away the veil that formerly surrounded the idea. We now know, viscerally that we CAN die and death might occur soon.

After the shock of the initial diagnosis has worn off and we now become somewhat accustomed to the idea, we begin to concentrate on treatment and how to conquer this disease. We also become aware of the secondary losses such as not being able to function in the way did formerly. If we are undergoing chemo-therapy or radiation, we probably will experience side-effects that incapacitate us at least for awhile. We now feel different from our friends and the non-cancer population. We are set apart and we need time to mourn our losses so that we can get through them and go on with our lives. Many of our relationships change, and we now take comfort in the sharing and trust in our support group where others nod their heads in affirmation as we speak. Some of our relationships become closer and we begin to evaluate everything in our lives using different criteria. For example: Am I living my life the way that I now choose? Am I making closer relationships, those that fit into my new self? What plans do I wish to carry out? If not now, when?

It takes time to reach these understandings, but in the meantime, we must live with the pain that has accompanied this disease. If we bury it, it will go somewhere else and affect us negatively. We can only get past it if we go through it.

SHARE had helped us do that, and the passage of time diminishes the rawness of the emotions.

Everyone's life contains loss and the way we get through it can open up doors to a better life.

## Regret and Redemption

Is the word "redemption" too strong to aptly describe what sometimes happens after we experience a diagnosis of cancer, or a lost breast, lost hair, diminished sex drive and diminished self-esteem? Perhaps, more importantly the loss of the fallible belief that we are immortal affects our lives in a most powerful and significant manner. The inevitability of death was always a reality, but its true meaning escaped us until the word "cancer" caused it to be an indelible part of our thinking and being.

Can that knowledge cripple us, or does it enlighten us and make us more conscious of the passage of time and the need to use time in a more meaningful manner; understanding how precious it is and how irretrievable? Does it defeat us or empower us? Is the love in our hearts deeper? Do we attach more meaning to our relationships? Do we pursue the plans we had always delayed or debated ad infinitum? And if so, do we wish we had never had cancer? YOU BET! We gained this knowledge the hard way. Would we have understood all this without the cancer? Perhaps, for the fortunate ones who have always lived with this understanding. But if this jolt helped us to lead our lives in a more fulfilling way, perhaps then, we have experienced some form of redemption. Only you can answer that question.

## Caregiver's Corner

When you are engaged in a death vigil for someone you love, the reality of that situation is obfuscated by your own denial and by various aspects and shades of hope. The smallest signs of improvement can be seen as a reprieve and the word "stable" takes on the significance of meaning "nothing is worse so we have more time." This concept is almost celebratory in tone.

The endless details of living; how towards the end the human being is reduced to the basic biological functions, occupies much of your thoughts. Eating becomes a complex activity. How nourished one feels when he eats! When you do know that someone you love will die, and knowing that this will probably happen within the next few months(you only know this in your head of course, because life is inconceivable without his presence, if only his physical presence) and the morphine and lack of oxygen to the brain take away a good deal of his persona he is still there. He is capable of looking at you, of being stroked and kissed, and you can still hear his voice.

How to be helpful without taking away his control, without making him feel diminished and without power? Is it possible to be the bridge to another person's life and not occasionally abuse power? How deep is the responsibility when another's life depends on you utterly and entirely? How do you avoid being petty and self-serving when it seems you have no life but his and you are aching for some fresh air? The details of your own life become unimportant and everything is gauged and measured in response to his needs. And the reality becomes the merging and melding of two people; the line between patient and caregiver is blurred.

You become expert at knowing all of his moods, his needs, his demands before he can even express them. This learning to anticipate in order to save his strength and increase his comfort becomes almost a science, but ultimately, it becomes an instinct based on your closeness and observation of him. His face and body are like road maps; you learn to read them accurately and carefully so that as he is opening his eyes, you are there with a smile on your face greeting him and welcoming him into the day. How many times you had to prepare that smile and fix it on your face before you entered the room!

You begin to memorize his face because deep within you, you know it will vanish soon. And when you try to imagine what life would be like without him, you invent a concept, a picture, but until death robs you of him, you can never really know. The look of him, the space he created, the utter emptiness and silence is beyond imagination. How your eyes long to see him; your ears to hear his voice; your hands to feel his skin, and there is nothing but a conjuring up of his being. You try to smell his clothing, handle his personal things, wear his socks just to feel connected, but it is all erased; a transitional object created to pretend that he is there. As time went on, he retreated from life as we had known it, and the pull of everyday existence lost its meaning for him, so that finally, I had to accept him where he was. My love underwent a metamorphosis and it became purified and intense and deep, removed of all the normal marital conflicts that have the luxury to exist when one is healthy. Then, gone is the resentment for the lack of my own life, but only the wish to prolong his life without pain.

When you are the one he wants to be his total caregiver, how do you make room for others who wish to demonstrate their love for him? You learn that you do not have to do everything yourself, you can ask for help; they needed to give it, and I needed to receive it. The wonderful thing about love is that there is always enough to go around.

At the very end, when there is no quality and his systems are shutting down, you begin to wish for the end ... for him and because the pain of watching this shutdown is too much to bear.

Somehow, your love has tapped depths and transformed you. It has released a new energy inside of you and will enable you to open your heart to others. Love gives meaning to life and when you are in the throes of caring for someone, remember that because when that person is gone, you will have to find an outlet for all of that love.

And the passage of time is different. Just as death came, I now know that it will come for all of us in its own time. Each day of life moves quickly, even the depressive and lonely ones. So, use that knowledge; enjoy each moment that you can, and when you are feeling empty inside, know that "this too shall pass."

Dedicated to the memory of Ed Miller

# Conclusion

Does a story ever really end? Even with death, the legacy lives on and affects the lives of others.

SHARE has been in existence for thirty years and this book describes the evolution of its first thirty It continues, ever-changing, but as with genes its makeup has marked its direction and possibilities.

This book has come from my heart, and although I have recorded the progress, emotions and reactions of hundreds of others, they represent a distillation of what I have learned from them.

It is possible that some of the details may not be accurate, and for that I apologize, but the lessons and feelings are authentic. We at SHARE have paved the way for so many others, and we are proud of the grass-roots origin of our organization. We have learned the value of supporting each other, and in receiving, our lives have become richer and deeper and have helped make us capable of giving back to others what we have received.

Establishing a reputation is a progressive thing: the layers of our foundation keep building and they produce an edifice which attests to what we represent It is impossible to measure one moment of understanding, some life-saving information given at just the right time, the bond of friendship and the desire to keep fighting and struggling and the comfort provided to us and our families and friends.

Is courage contagious? A very difficult question. Having associated with so many courageous people who face difficult treatment and the possibility of imminent death, I wonder whether some of that spirit can rub off on others. What does courage in this context actually mean? I know it does not mean the elimination of sadness or feelings of hopelessness and despair but despite these feelings are we able to acknowledge what lies ahead of us and decide to face those forces and do our best to hold on to a glimmer of hope (if that means diminishing pain or saying "goodbye" to loved ones)? Does having courage mean we have to pretend to those around us that we can handle this and do our utmost not to share our innermost frightened feelings with others? In support groups, we are able to speak honestly and to receive validation from the other members who are going through a similar experience.

What effect does courage have on those around us? Does it make the rest of us feel inadequate?

The answers to these questions vary. My reaction is that courage is not contagious but it is certainly inspirational. And in the end, that may help us lead our lives in a way that inspires others.

And so, it is hoped that this book will underscore what we are all capable of achieving: an appreciation of life and love and the feeling of being part of a community where our connection to cancer and to each other connects us all.

# History of SHARE

1976- SHARE'S grass roots organization began with a radio announcement by Arlene Francis on her radio show. Dr. Eugene Thiessen, a
concerned breast specialist invited women with breast cancer to form
a support group dealing with emotional and psychosocial issues.
About twelve women responded to the ad.

1977- SHARE incorporated as a non-profit organization, staffed exclusively by volunteers.

1978- Large meetings, open to the public, were held inviting experts in the
breast cancer field to speak.

1979- Breast Cancer Hotline became operational. Support groups started
meeting in Queens.

1983- Wellness programs were introduced to explore relationships between
stress and breast cancer.

1986- The first SHARE office was opened through the efforts of Barbara
Kronman, who served as Executive Director from 1987-1989.

1987- SHARE published its first newsletter for program participants and
contributors. Our first support group for metastatic women was
started by Roberta Huffnagel

1989- We move to our own office.

1991-  The first SHARE-A-Walk was held, raising the public's awareness
about breast cancer and raising $125,000 to help support SHARE'S
services. It was initiated by Sally Berg, who had served as Co-Direc-
tor since 1989.

1992-  Spanish language hotline was introduced. Latina support groups
were held at six community sites in the four boroughs of New York
City.

1993-  SHARE—A-Walk drew more than thirty-five hundred participants
including Bella Abzug, Diane Sawyer and Linda Ellerbee.

Alice Yaker became Executive Director, and Harlem SHARE
started.

1994-  Volunteers answered more than five thousand hotline calls.

1995-  Ovarian Cancer Program began its first support group in New York.

1996-  Ovarian Cancer program hotline was established.
The Bereavement Program was started including support groups and
an annual Memorial Ceremony.

1997-  SHARE'S hotline volunteers answered more than seven thousand
calls in nine languages.

1998-  SHARE survivors had dialogues with medical students and residents
at N. Y.U. on communication, end-of-life issues and cultural diversity.

SHARE reached more than thirty thousand women, men and children.

1999-  SHARE'S website was launched

2000-  New partnership formed with ST. Vincent's Comprehensive Cancer
Center.

2001- SHARE'S installation of our Donor Recognition Wall.

Expansion of the New Jersey affiliate.

2004- SHARE hosted its first annual "Second Helping of Life", a toasting event to benefit SHARE, featuring New York City's top women chefs.

2005- Governor Pataki awarded SHARE a Breast Cancer and Education Award for a non-profit organization.

2005 Attorney General of New York awarded us a grant for a New York State Ovarian Hotline (in conjunction with the American Cancer society).

A SHARE Emeritus Board is formed.

# About the Author

After a radical mastectomy in 1975, Lee Miller became a founding member of an organization called SHARE founded by Dr. Eugene Thiessen. She has consistently played a very active part in designing programs such as facilitation and hotline training, patient/doctor communication, and the bereavement program. She was President of the Board of Directors for eight years and is a member of the Emeritus Board.

Her background of social work, law, counseling and psycho-therapy have consistently shown a core interest in advocacy for the student, teacher, client and patient.

She served for three years on Surgeon-General Koop's Task Force on Self-Help and Public Health and that experience affirmed her belief that peer support changed people's lives. She also served on the Board of Directors of the New York Self-Help Clearinghouse for several years.

However, her role as mother, grandmother and widow have deepened her life thus creating a richer tapestry for her work.

She is proud to be part of this not-for profit organization, which has always been responsive to the ever-growing requests for programs and projects and has helped so many women weather the storms of cancer with dignity and courage.

978-0-595-42981-3
0-595-42981-5